Technology and Competency-Oriented Learning

Lior Naamati-Schneider · Dorit Alt

Technology and Competency-Oriented Learning

Effective Methods for Training the Next Cohort of Healthcare Managers

Springer

Lior Naamati-Schneider
Health Systems Management Department
Hadassah Academic College
Jerusalem, Israel

Dorit Alt
Faculty of Education and Teaching
Tel Hai College
Qiryat Shemona, Israel

ISBN 978-981-97-5770-1 ISBN 978-981-97-5771-8 (eBook)
https://doi.org/10.1007/978-981-97-5771-8

This Springer imprint is published by the registered company Springer Nature Singapore Pte Ltd.
The registered company address is: 152 Beach Road, #21-01/04 Gateway East, Singapore 189721, Singapore

Contents

About the Authors

Dr. Lior Naamati-Schneider is a senior lecturer and researcher in the Health Systems Management Department at Hadassah Academic College, Israel. Her research focuses on health policy, healthcare management, and medical education, with an emphasis on adaptation processes within the healthcare system. She examines individual, organizational, and systemic aspects to meet the evolving needs of the healthcare market. With over 25 years of experience in both teaching and practical management, she has contributed to innovative, technology-based learning environments aimed at enhancing students' lifelong learning skills.

Prof. Dorit Alt serves as the dean of the Faculty of Education and Teaching at Tel-Hai College in Israel. Her area of expertise lies in the development, implementation, and evaluation of future-oriented, technology-enhanced, and competency-based learning. Central to her studies is the design and evaluation of innovative learning environments that aim to enhance learners' abilities in achieving personal well-being, social sensitivity, and economic and occupational prosperity amidst social and global changes. She has authored research papers in leading scientific journals, and her research has earned her a prominent standing in the scientific international arena.

Chapter 1
Preface

The twenty-first century is marked by a rapid accumulation of knowledge together with numerous and profound changes, developments and advances in complex technologies that have begun to exert control over many spheres of our lives. These widespread changes have also had an impact on healthcare systems across the globe and on the medical profession as a whole (Laprise, 2023). Consequently, healthcare systems and professionals must adapt to be able to cope with the constant changes and new challenges posed by this dynamic era (Deshpande et al., 2023; Naamati-Schneider, 2020, 2022; Naamati-Schneider & Salvatore, 2023). These challenges are also linked to the growing use of advanced technology and artificial intelligence, as well as to alterations in the nature and scope of the health management profession (Ali et al., 2023; Manne & Kantheti, 2021). These trends have emerged in the context of other changes, among them the introduction of new regulations and reforms, increased longevity, and various geographic, demographic, economic, and political changes (Figueroa et al., 2019). Moreover, societies across the globe are becoming increasingly diverse (Weech-Maldonado et al., 2018), thus affecting the extensive ecosystem within which healthcare systems and organizations must operate.

Market conditions in the medical field are also characterized by diminishing resources. These conditions have generated a chronic and constantly growing discrepancy between rising health expenditures and limited funding, placing pressure and overload on health systems. Moreover, extreme crisis situations such as those experienced during the COVID-19 outbreak pose a threat to the future sustainability, survival and stability of health systems worldwide (Naamati-Schneider & Salvatore, 2023; OECD, 2020).

To be able to provide high-quality health services, health systems and organizations across the globe must adopt appropriate managerial and business behavior patterns and adapt to change at all levels: macro, meso, and micro (Ginter et al., 2018). Consequently, health management that encompasses a comprehensive understanding of business management and of the intricate nature of health systems has become an essential element of healthcare. (Raftery et al, 2022).

L. Naamati-Schneider and D. Alt, *Technology and Competency-Oriented Learning*,
https://doi.org/10.1007/978-981-97-5771-8_1

Accordingly, managers and staff members in the healthcare system must acquire a set of updated twenty-first century skills (21CS) that will enable them to cope with new and unstable situations. These skills must cover three core domains of competence: cognitive, intrapersonal, and interpersonal. Such capabilities are becoming an essential and inseparable part of the array of tasks that twenty-first century healthcare managers must be able to perform (American College of Healthcare Executives, 2022; Tindowen et al., 2017). In response to this need, the healthcare education system must develop curricula to teach the required skills to those studying healthcare management and other health professions. These educational programs must help their students adapt to new situations during the course of their studies and throughout their professional lives. Nevertheless, although this notion has become accepted worldwide, very few educational systems have integrated these skills into their policy. This is mainly because many higher education systems continue to adhere to back-to-basics educational methods that hamper the diffusion of competency-based learning methods into educational systems (Nehring et al., 2019; Vista, 2020).

In view of the importance of this issue and the need for healthcare management professionals to assimilate these abilities, and considering the scant research conducted in this field, this book seeks to propose innovative, technology-enabled teaching and learning methods aimed at fostering the relevant skills among managers in the healthcare system. Under the framework of competency-based learning, these methods aim to transition from the traditional focus on recitation and memorization to constructivist approaches that enhance students' skills through interactive techniques (European Commission, 2018; Shorey et al., 2019).

This book adopts an integrative approach to examining healthcare organizations and professionals that encompasses all levels of the system: macro, meso, and micro. It explores how processes of change affect these three levels while highlighting the essential set of skills needed for navigating these transformations successfully. Drawing on the 21CS taxonomy developed by the National Research Council (2012), each chapter of this volume focuses on a specific skill relevant to healthcare managers. The text demonstrates how educators can use competency-based learning approaches to foster these skills, with Fig. 1.1 providing a mapping sentence to present the scope and organization of a book. A mapping sentence is a structured statement that outlines the main themes and concepts covered in each chapter, providing a clear and logical overview of the material. This approach helps readers to quickly understand the scope and organization of the book.

The book seeks to provide valuable insights into the development of competency-based learning approaches and specific learning and instructional activities that can enhance 21CS among healthcare management students. It also strives to enhance our understanding of how to help healthcare managers develop lifelong learning skills effectively and at an early stage of their training. Such abilities will position these professionals to be able to contend with the diverse needs of the digital age and with changing and dynamic technological and medical knowledge. This book may also serve as a valuable and up-to-date reference for healthcare and pedagogical research. It is suited for a wide audience, including healthcare students and faculty members, policymakers, and higher education curriculum designers.

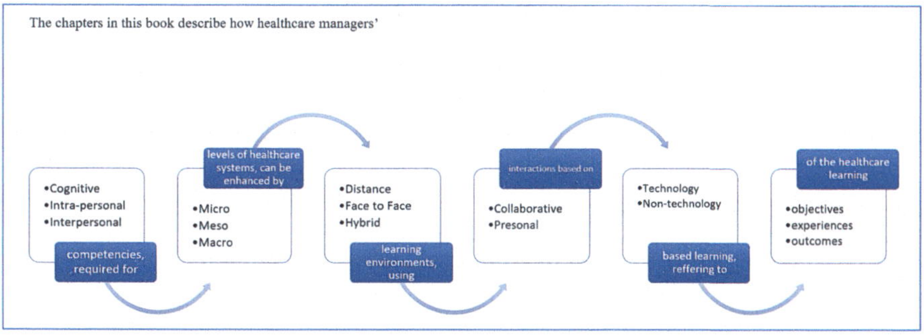

Fig. 1.1 A mapping sentence describing the contexts of the chapters in this volume

The book is divided into eleven chapters, organized around the three fundamental domains of competence: cognitive, intrapersonal, and interpersonal.

Part I: Adapting to a Changing Ecosystem: Environmental Change and the Need to Adapt

Chapter 2: The Complex and Ever-Changing Environment of Healthcare Systems: Characteristics and Future Challenges

Chapter 2 serves as an initial introduction to the dynamic nature of global healthcare systems by focusing on the environment of healthcare organizations and the transformative changes they have undergone in recent decades. The chapter describes the macro, meso and micro levels of healthcare systems and examines the unfolding processes of change and their ongoing effects within these levels over time. Furthermore, the chapter addresses the limitations, issues and challenges associated with implementing these change processes and emphasizes the ongoing need for adaptive measures and effective management, including appropriate training. Such efforts are crucial for enabling systems and the individuals within them to navigate current and future challenges effectively. Indeed, fostering their ability to adapt within the evolving professional and managerial landscape will ultimately contribute to preparing them for the world of tomorrow.

Chapter 3: Competency-Based Learning and Real-World Performance in Health Management Professions

Chapter 3 begins by drawing upon the 21CS taxonomy proposed by the National Research Council (2012) and on other contemporary classifications related to health management. It examines learning experiences that can help students effectively acquire 21CS, with specific focus on competency-based learning approaches implemented by faculty members. Competency-based learning is an educational approach that focuses on the outcomes of learning rather than the process. In competency-based learning, the emphasis is on students demonstrating mastery of specific skills or competencies, which are clearly defined and measurable. The chapter explores the impact of these competency-based learning approaches on students' perceived cognitive, intrapersonal, and interpersonal 21CS. The chapter provides a comprehensive definition of 21CS and emphasizes the increasing importance of these skills in the academic literature and on the job market. It also elucidates the concept of competency-based learning and showcases how such methods have been utilized and researched within the context of health management curricula.

Part II: Cognitive Competencies

Chapter 4: Using Digital Concept Maps to Promote Argumentation Skills and Epistemological Beliefs Among Healthcare Management Students

Chapter 4 illustrates the effective application of constructivist pedagogy to problem-solving, with a specific focus on using argumentation in distance learning contexts. It describes a course for undergraduate health system management students in which a traditional face-to-face activity was replaced by an online-based argumentation-based learning activity during the COVID-19 pandemic. The chapter explores the key challenges and potential opportunities offered by this novel approach that incorporates an online argumentation-based learning activity with digital concept mapping (CM) to enhance learning. The primary objective of this approach is to foster lifelong learning skills such as high-order thinking, critical thinking, and problem-solving abilities among health management students.

Chapter 5: Cultivating Future Thinking, Creativity, and Innovation through E-Poster Engagement: Essential Competencies for Contemporary Healthcare Managers

Chapter 5 explores the role of future problem-solving programs in fostering learner creativity, particularly by enhancing crucial skills for flexible thinking together with creative, fluent and innovative problem-solving methods. The chapter demonstrates how the Future Problem Solving (FPS) program was used in health management courses. Students participated in a six-step program in which they addressed future challenges and proposed practical solutions. Implementation of the FPS program encouraged participants to generate innovative and diverse solutions for complex problems, identify unknown factors, and establish connections among seemingly unrelated ideas. The chapter describes the FPS technique in detail and discusses its contribution to health management students' awareness of creative and innovative ideas and techniques that can be used in health professions.

Chapter 6: Moving Toward Digital Transformation: Building eHealth Literacy Skills Among Healthcare Managers

Chapter 6 focuses on the process of integrating medical literacy skills within healthcare organizations and among healthcare managers and professionals by examining various projects aimed at cultivating these skills. The chapter describes a practical application of faculty guidance in online healthcare management education and discusses its impact on students' eHealth Literacy skills, while highlighting the effectiveness of this approach and its contribution to skill development. The described program incorporates methodologies such as future case studies and e-posters to facilitate acquisition of these skills. Additionally, the chapter introduces an instructional e-model specifically designed for higher education and aimed at enhancing students' digital literacy skills.

Part III—IntraPersonal Competencies

Chapter 7: Healthcare Management Students' Self-Regulation Skills: Helping Students Become Proactive Learners

Chapter 7 highlights the critical role of self-regulated learning (SRL) in enabling healthcare professionals to adapt to the rapidly changing healthcare market (Bransen et al., 2020). The chapter describes a case in which SRL was integrated into the medical curriculum and highlights the importance of SRL in promoting proactive learning behaviors, enhancing metacognitive skills, and increasing motivation.

The use of reflective journal writing as an educational tool in medical education constitutes a major focus of this chapter. This approach is proposed as a strategy for fostering SRL among students to facilitate deeper engagement with educational material and reflection on their learning journey. Additionally, it is important for the development of personal identity and enhancing the ability to influence practice. The chapter suggests that by encouraging such reflective practices, medical education can more effectively prepare students for the complexities and challenges they will face in their professional healthcare roles. The overarching goal is to develop a workforce that is not only professionally skilled, but also adaptable, resilient and equipped for continuous learning in the ever-evolving landscape of the healthcare setting.

Chapter 8: Ethical Judgment and Ethical Leadership In Healthcare Management Education

Chapter 8 examines the implications of changes in the global ecosystem on the ethical aspects of the healthcare market, focusing on strategic and technological shifts. These changes have engendered the need to exercise ethical judgment, construct an ethical code for medical management, and develop ethical leadership in the health field. The chapter describes various intervention programs in diverse settings for promoting and developing these competencies at all levels of training, from the onset of professional studies through professional training within the healthcare organizations themselves. Inculcation and development of ethical judgment among healthcare systems managers and healthcare organizations will help generate trust among the various parts of the system, including patients, and will contribute to strengthening the values of equity and quality in the health system.

Part IV: Interpersonal Competencies

Chapter 9: Managerial Leadership in Healthcare Systems

Chapter 9 explores the differences and overlaps between medical leadership and management by examining various models and forms of medical leadership, as well as intervention programs designed to cultivate leadership skills in different health sectors in both academic and healthcare organization contexts. The chapter traces the educational progress of leadership training, from students at the beginning of their educational journey to experienced senior managers. It also highlights the evolving dynamics of change within the healthcare system and its managerial leadership, both now and in the future, and identifies key educational strategies for fostering effective medical management leadership. The chapter emphasizes the importance of timely planning, awareness of potential challenges and the development of leadership and management skills in healthcare. This approach seeks to prepare professionals in advance and to plan change processes strategically, thereby ensuring system stability and improving patient care.

Chapter 10: Customer/Patient Service Orientation: Nurturing Service Competencies in Healthcare Systems

Chapter 10 offers an extensive examination of the implications of environmental changes on service orientation across the three levels discussed in the book: macro, meso and micro. It investigates how to cultivate a service orientation and what competencies are required at each level. The chapter sheds light on the transformations in the healthcare system with respect to customer service orientation and patient-centered care. Furthermore, it outlines essential educational practices aimed at training the healthcare workforce at the managerial and clinical levels to adapt to these changes. To further elucidate the principles of this approach and to establish a solid foundation for driving and implementing change, the chapter describes the use of methodological tools and intervention plans among students and staff in healthcare management. This approach ensures the continuity of high-quality care and services while enhancing the efficiency and stability of the healthcare system over the long term.

Chapter 11: Online Collaborative Padlet-Mediated Learning in Health Management Studies

Chapter 11 demonstrates the effectiveness of online collaborative learning (OCL) by exemplifying the use of Padlet as a digital platform for interactive collaboration in health management education. Developing collaboration skills is essential for healthcare professionals, who often work in diverse teams of people from different backgrounds. Introducing OCL environments early in professional training can help nurture these skills. The widespread adoption of OCL pedagogies across all levels of education, from undergraduate studies to professional development, is believed to offer significant benefits for the healthcare system and its patients. This is particularly important considering the practical nature of work in the healthcare industry.

The chapter focuses on analyzing students' perceptions of their experiences with Padlet-facilitated OCL by seeking to understand how they perceived the activity and its implications. Content analysis is used to identify themes and patterns regarding students' perceptions of the newly designed activity. The core objective of this chapter is to understand the advantages of Padlet as a collaborative learning tool that facilitates the development of teamwork abilities, collaborative decision-making skills, and adaptability to changes in the learning environment.

Chapter 12: Integrating AI into Healthcare: Implications for Medical Education and Management

Chapter 12 aims to examine the various potential applications of AI tools in healthcare administration and medical care at all levels of the healthcare system. It emphasizes the challenges and obstacles associated with implementing AI in medical settings. Indeed, addressing these issues is crucial in preparing for the forthcoming changes. The discussion also focuses on the integration of AI tools into education and training programs in higher education and at medical institutions. It emphasizes the need for healthcare managers and professionals to develop a new set of competencies that will enable them to adapt to the evolving landscape. These competencies will allow them to embrace and adjust to the upcoming expected use of AI in healthcare. Furthermore, the chapter provides an overview of current innovative initiatives aimed at implementing these competencies in academic and organizational healthcare settings

Epilogue

This chapter highlights the transformative impacts of the changing ecosystem and technological advancements on healthcare systems. It underscores the critical need for competency-based education to prepare healthcare professionals for ongoing changes. By focusing on lifelong learning and adaptable management skills, the chapter provides strategic recommendations for educators and healthcare leaders at macro, meso, and micro levels. These strategies aim to enhance the efficiency, quality, and stability of healthcare systems, ensuring they are well-equipped to navigate future challenges and improve patient outcomes.

References

Ali, O., Abdelbaki, W., Shrestha, A., Elbasi, E., Alryalat, M. A. A., & Dwivedi, Y. K. (2023). A systematic literature review of artificial intelligence in the healthcare sector: Benefits, challenges, methodologies, and functionalities. *Journal of Innovation & Knowledge, 8*(1), 100333. https://doi.org/10.1016/j.jik.2023.100333

American College of Healthcare Executives. (2022). ACHE healthcare executive 2022 competencies assessment tool. https://www.ache.org/-/media/ache/careerresource-center/cat-2022.pdf

Bransen, D., Govaerts, M. J., Sluijsmans, D. M., & Driessen, E. W. (2020). Beyond the self: The role of co-regulation in medical students' self-regulated learning. *Medical Education, 54*(3), 234–241. https://doi.org/10.1111/medu.14018

Deshpande, N., Arora, V. M., Vollbrecht, H., Meltzer, D. O., & Press, V. (2023). EHealth literacy and patient portal use and attitudes: Cross-sectional observational study. *JMIR Human Factors, 10*, e40105. https://doi.org/10.2196/40105

European Commission. (2018). Commission staff working document accompanying the document proposal for a council recommendation on key competences for lifelong learning. https://ec.europa.eu/

Figueroa, C. A., Harrison, R., Chauhan, A., & Meyer, L. (2019). Priorities and challenges for health leadership and workforce management globally: A rapid review. *BMC Health Services Research, 19*(1), 1–11. https://doi.org/10.1186/s12913-019-4080-7

Ginter, P. M., Duncan, W. J., & Swayne, L. E. (2018). *The strategic management of health care organisations*. Wiley.

Laprise, C. (2023). It's time to take a sustainable approach to health care in the face of the challenges of the 21st century. *One Health, 16*, 100510.

Manne, R., & Kantheti, S. C. (2021). Application of artificial intelligence in healthcare: Chances and challenges. *Current Journal of Applied Science and Technology, 40*(6), 78–89. https://doi.org/10.9734/cjast/2021/v40i631320

Naamati Schneider, L. (2020). Strategic management as an adaptation to changes in the ecosystems of public hospitals in Israel. *Israel Journal of Health Policy Research 9*. https://doi.org/10.1186/s13584-020-00424-y

Naamati-Schneider, L. (2022). Intraorganization conflicts of interest in hospitals adapting to a changing ecosystem. *Journal of Health Organization and Management, 36*(3), 265–278. https://doi.org/10.1108/JHOM-09-2021-0325

Naamati-Schneider, L., & Salvatore, F. P. (2023). Sustainability for healthcare organisations and systems: Cultivating strategy and governance processes for a better future. In D. Vrontis, A. Thrassou, L. Efthymiou, Y. Weber, S. M. R. Shams, & E. Tsoukatos, (Eds.), *Business for sustainability. Volume I: Strategic avenues and managerial approaches* (pp. 227–248). Springer. https://doi.org/10.1007/978-3-031-37361-9_11

National Research Council. (2012). In J. W. Pellegrino & M. L. Hilton (Eds.), *Education for life and work: Developing transferable knowledge and skills in the 21st Century.* Committee on Defining Deeper Learning and 21st Century Skills, Board on Testing and Assessment and Board on Science Education, Division of Behavioral and Social Sciences and Education. The National Academies Press. Retrieved from https://www.nap.edu/catalog/13398/education-for-life-and-work-developing-transferable-knowledge-and-skills.

Nehring, J. H., Charner-Laird, M., & Szczesiul, S. A. (2019). Redefining excellence: Teaching in transition, from test performance to 21st century skills. *NASSP Bulletin, 103*(1), 5–31. https://doi.org/10.1177/0192636519830772

OECD. (2020). *Organisation for economic cooperation and development global health spending data.* Retrieved from https://data.oecd.org/healthres/health-spending.htm,.

Raftery, C., Sassenberg, A. M., & Bamford-Wade, A. (2022). Business acumen for nursing leaders: An exploratory qualitative study. *Journal of Nursing Management, 30*(7), 2681–2688. https://doi.org.mgs.hac.ac.il/10.1111/jonm.13672

Shorey, S., Lau, T. C., Lau, S. T., & Ang, E. (2019). Entrustable professional activities in health care education: A scoping review. *Medical Education, 53*(8), 766–777.

Tindowen, D. J. C., Bassig, J. M., & Cagurangan, J. A. (2017). Twenty-first-century skills of alternative learning system learners. *Sage Open, 7*(3). https://doi.org/10.1177/2158244017726116

Vista, A. (2020). Data-driven identification of skills for the future: 21st-century skills for the 21st-century workforce. *SAGE Open, 10*(2), 2158244020915904. https://doi.org/10.1111/medu.13879

Weech-Maldonado, R., Dreachslin, J. L., Epané, J. P., Gail, J., Gupta, S., & Wainio, J. A. (2018). Hospital cultural competency as a systematic organizational intervention: Key findings from the national center for healthcare leadership diversity demonstration project. *Health Care Management Review, 43*(1), 30–41. https://doi.org/10.1097/HMR.0000000000000128

Part I
Adapting to a Changing Ecosystem: Environmental Change and the Need to Adapt

Chapter 2
The Complex and Ever-Changing Environment of Healthcare Systems: Characteristics and Future Challenges

Abstract Global healthcare systems are undergoing dynamic transformations, necessitating a closer look at the changes within healthcare organizations over recent decades. This chapter delves into these shifts, examining the macro, meso, and micro levels of healthcare systems and the ongoing processes of change. It addresses the limitations, issues, and challenges in implementing these changes, underscoring the need for adaptive measures and effective management. Essential efforts, including targeted training, are vital for systems and individuals to navigate current and future challenges, ultimately preparing them for the evolving professional and managerial landscape of tomorrow.

Introduction

The past few decades have been marked by significant changes brought about by technological advancements, automation, and the development of digital and virtual worlds. Driven by creativity, innovation, and cooperation, these changes have had far-reaching effects on the global economy. This resulting new reality demands increased professionalism in various fields, with greater focus on capabilities for solving unstructured problems and effective information analysis (World Economic Forum, 2015). The broad consensus today is that these environmental changes are altering reality and presenting new challenges to people in many areas.

Attempts are being made to characterize and define these changes so that systems and those working within them can adapt to the changing demands. Indeed, people are beginning to understand that today's reality is marked by volatility, uncertainty, complexity, and ambiguity (VUCA). This concept, derived from the military, is now commonly used in the field of management in recognition of the increasingly complex organizational challenges in the current era (Otter, 2019).

The repercussions of this reality, particularly the worldwide need to cope with VUCA and the extensive and complex challenges posed by this reality, have also affected global healthcare systems and the various organizations that comprise them (Cernega et al., 2024; Counte et al., 2019; WHO, 2019; Worley & Jules, 2020). This

L. Naamati-Schneider and D. Alt, *Technology and Competency-Oriented Learning*,
https://doi.org/10.1007/978-981-97-5771-8_2

chapter describes the environment of these health organizations and the changes they have undergone over the past several decades. It also describes the division of healthcare systems into macro, meso, and micro levels, reviews the processes of change within healthcare systems over the past decades and examines the repercussions at all three levels. The chapter also discusses the limitations, problems, and challenges in adopting these change processes and the ongoing need to adapt and manage them. It explains that providing suitable training will enable both healthcare systems and individuals to better cope with current and future challenges from both the professional and the managerial perspectives to help them adapt to the world of the future.

Healthcare Systems Within a Complex and Ever-Changing Environment

The following section examines changes in the global and local healthcare ecosystem. Within this framework, we discuss general external changes that apply across the globe and directly or indirectly affect healthcare systems, as well as local changes. We also examine extreme changes, such as the crisis emerging from the COVID-19 pandemic and the impact of these changes on healthcare systems as organizations, on healthcare professionals, and on patients.

Over the past decades, healthcare systems worldwide and the organizations and people working under their auspices have had to cope with extensive and complex challenges caused by various local and global factors. In the context of healthcare systems, the most predominant reasons for these changes include demographic, technological, economic, and political factors that affect the wide-ranging ecosystem within which they operate (Counte et al., 2019; WHO, 2019).

At the same time, the need for healthcare systems is on the rise due to increased life expectancy accompanied by an ageing population and an increase in the incidence of chronic disease. Furthermore, growing awareness of health issues among the world's population has resulted in a mounting demand for and greater consumption of healthcare products, as evidenced in an increase in the amount and availability of medical services and modern medical technology. Yet these additional needs have not been accompanied by any increased allotment of financial resources (Papanicolas et al., 2018).

This situation has led to an inherent gap within healthcare systems between mounting health expenditures and limited funding. This gap is growing from day to day and must be curbed and managed. Indeed, it is undoubtedly one of the most challenging problems currently confronting healthcare services, posing a threat to their future sustainability, survival, and stability (Naamati-Schneider & Salvatore, 2023; OECD, 2020).

The measures necessary to cope with this gap alongside additional changes and regulatory and financial pressures have created a tumultuous, challenging, and competitive environment within healthcare systems, one that their leaders must cope with in order to survive (Counte et al., 2019; Ginter et al., 2018; Naamati-Schneider, 2020).

Healthcare systems and organizations worldwide must change and adapt themselves to these processes of change that are having an impact on the different areas and levels of the system. In response, healthcare organizations have been compelled to change their managerial, organizational, and financial behavior (Bin-Nun, 2019; Naamati-Schneider, 2021, 2023).

The outbreak of the COVID-19 pandemic in December 2019 significantly increased the pressure on healthcare systems and organizations due to the immediate need to cope with the emerging health crisis and provide an answer for patients. These systems were forced to deal with an unfamiliar and highly contagious disease, cope with overload and burnout, reduce the availability of elective medical procedures, and delay additional medical activities (Argenziano et al., 2020). This situation seriously damaged the financial stability of healthcare organizations such as clinics and hospitals, which were forced to decrease the extent of their activities, lengthen the amount of time patients waited for treatments, and deal with cutbacks in human resources, all of which had a detrimental impact upon their income and reputation (Ron & Weiss, 2020; Zangrandi et al., 2020).

These difficulties impelled healthcare organizations and systems to adapt to the changing environment by adopting, developing, and implementing immediate and creative medical and financial solutions. Hence, the COVID-19 crisis constituted a significant incentive for growth and for adopting various medical, managerial, and technological changes aimed at coping with market distress, uncertainty and competition in order to survive (Naamati-Schneider & Zaks, 2022).

Adopting and assimilating change processes within healthcare organizations and systems involved, among other things, instituting technological changes that generated additional secondary changes, among them changes in level of care and medical services and changes at the organizational and managerial levels. These changes provoked other solutions for coping with the damage brought about by the crisis (Bar, 2020). Thus the financial distress of health organizations and their increasing need to show profitability inspired horizontal cooperation within and outside the system. For example, cooperation began to flourish with private startup and high-tech companies, some of which were redesigned to meet the changing needs. Such instances of cooperation are an example of the changing health market and its managerial and public character. These rapid changes and the variety of the solutions proposed stimulate organizational changes and affect the entire system and its demands (Naamati-Schneider & Zaks, 2022).

One example of this overall impact is the digital transformation of all parts of the system. The digital transformation processes characteristic of the twenty-first century are part of the fourth industrial revolution. One of the areas marked by extensive digital changes is healthcare (Kraus et al., 2021; Marques & Ferreira, 2020; Schwab, 2017).

These processes of digital transformation within healthcare systems and organizations are significant in that they have paved the way for new treatment and management solutions. The digital technologies being assimilated into healthcare have led to increased efficiency and improved performance, while ensuring optimal utilization of resources. Through appropriate use of these digital change processes, organizations are striving to create stability and sustainability (Marques & Ferreira, 2020; Naamati-Schneider & Salvatore, 2023).

The digital transformation processes in healthcare systems and organizations are extensive, encompassing diverse areas such as diagnosis, treatment, research, service, and accessibility. For example, the assimilation of artificial intelligence and big data in the analysis of medical information has facilitated research, diagnosis and treatment, led to the establishment of global databases, and enabled the use of robotics and technologies for distance diagnosis and treatment, personalized medicine, telemedicine, digital services, treatment continuity, and computerized patient file management (Marques & Ferreira, 2020; Kraus et al., 2021).

Similar changes are also occurring in patient environments. Digital tools and applications have made medical research, general databases, personal medical information, and services more accessible and available. Yet at the same time, these tools also result in a rise in the demand for medical services, and this increased demand causes new difficulties and obstacles for both the system and the patients (Bozorgmehr et al., 2020; Ricciardi et al., 2019).

The UN 2030 Agenda for Sustainable Development launched in 2015 outlines these changes, along with the need to adapt healthcare systems across the globe to the world of the future (United Nations, 2016). This document sets out 17 goals for sustainable development in various areas. Section 2.3 is devoted to the goal of good health and well-being. Its objective is to preserve health and provide healthcare services to the population while adopting changes and making adaptations within the overall system of healthcare organizations and those working within them. This goal entails adopting organizational, perceptual, cultural, and managerial processes of change, together with the technological transformations discussed previously, throughout the system and within the various organizations that comprise it. To do so, healthcare systems must be receptive to extensive development and investment in changes and environmental adaptation processes (Tjahjono et al., 2017).

An inseparable feature of modifying the environment of healthcare organizations and adapting them to processes of change involves changing how system managers are defined and characterized. The distinction between management and medical roles is frequently unclear, necessitating the development of hybrid multidisciplinary roles that combine medical and managerial knowledge while developing and integrating a variety of soft skills and abilities that the current period demands (Arora et al., 2010).

Healthcare organizations that were once oriented to the caregivers and to the organization itself have begun to place the patient at the center. They have acknowledged the need to assimilate changes that will transform them into customer/patient-centered organizations, while adopting competitive business and marketing strategies (Naamati-Schneider, 2020, 2021). These changes pose numerous problems arising from various conflict of interests within the system, among them a clash of ideals between the pure and principled world of medicine and the need to make business and marketing decisions. These decisions are often incompatible with the values, beliefs, and behavior that previously characterized the medical world (Naamati-Schneider, 2022). Making these necessary changes has affected the conduct of health-care systems and organizations and has posed multi-system, organizational, and personal challenges, among them the need to develop specific capabilities suitable to the changing healthcare environment, such as flexibility, creativity, and leadership to initiate and assimilate changes (Reis, 2019; Reis et al., 2013). To develop the necessary processes of change, the healthcare system must adopt changes across the board that will enable it to provide high-quality health services within the existing market limitations.

Three Levels of the Healthcare System: Micro, Meso, and Macro

In this section, we explain the levels of analysis within the healthcare system in the context of three levels used to define any social system. Each level of analysis is important for understanding and addressing issues and they are often interconnected and interdependent. The most comprehensive level of analysis is the macro level, which examines wide-ranging social structures and institutions such as governments, international organizations, and large corporations. The meso level is an intermediate level of analysis and focuses on smaller communities and organizations. The micro level is the smallest level of analysis and focuses on individual behavior and interpersonal relationships. We now examine each level in the context of health issues.

The macro level refers to the overall system. It includes all processes, policies and objectives and is responsible for determining the order of priorities within the framework of demographic, economic, technological, and political changes common to all healthcare systems across the world (Figueroa et al., 2019).

Implementation of global changes at the macro level must also consider issues such as demands concerning the quantity and quality of medical care services as a result of the population's growing consumerism and medical literacy (Potluri & Johnson, 2023). These issues exert additional pressure and require the healthcare system to attempt to meet patient demands that are often difficult to fulfill (Iliffe & Manthorpe, 2020). These patient demands are exacerbated by underbudgeting conditions marking healthcare systems worldwide (Hall et al., 2018).

The meso level incorporates management policies and planning strategies at the organizational/strategic level. These include adapting the organization to current needs and making strategic managerial and functional decisions, such as budget management, purchasing, work processes, and human resource management. For example, the need to make organizational changes and develop an organizational culture that encourages flexibility and intra-organizational and intra-disciplinary cooperation has increased in recent years. Making such changes is hindered by bureaucratic processes, cultural and managerial hierarchy, opposition to change, and the demand to provide extensive and high-quality health services at a low cost (Azzolini et al., 2018; Nilsen et al., 2020). This complex situation has compelled the healthcare system to fill most managerial positions with medical professionals who have not received proper managerial training, thus creating conflicts of interest and internal complexities that are not supported by the organization (Mercer et al., 2018; Naamati-Schneider, 2021, 2022). Another change at this level is the shift to a more service-oriented and customer-centered orientation. This shift, which has broad implications at all levels of management and care, finds expression in a new emphasis toward catering to clients' interests, needs and expectations and offering suitable services accordingly, i.e., relating to patients as customers (Bruno et al., 2017). The result is that health organizations have begun offering a wide variety of customer-centered services and products. This new emphasis alters the focus at the organizational and treatment levels, with patients becoming more and more active and assuming greater control over decision-making processes.

Healthcare organizations have begun using this altered focus to distinguish themselves as innovative organizations adapted to their clients and the market. This enables them to establish a high value chain for the organization and provides them with a relative competitive advantage in a highly competitive market (Ginter et al., 2018).

This transformation to a customer-centered, service-oriented organization together with the notion of relating to patients as customers and the repercussions of this change upon the organization's business and marketing activities are all foreign to healthcare organizations. Indeed, these processes often contradict the characteristics and terminology previously acceptable in the medical world. For this reason, dealing with these changes on a regular basis sometimes constitutes a hardship and challenge for the system and its staff (Naamati-Schneider, 2022). Adopting these changes on an organizational level therefore requires assimilation and adaptation strategies as well as training staff and managers to adopt changes optimally and effectively by teaching them to develop a variety of abilities that were not required previously.

The micro level refers to the individual managers and members of the medical staff. In recent years the job descriptions of doctors/managers within health organizations have undergone extensive changes (Figueroa et al., 2019). These changes have led to blurred boundaries, an absence of job descriptions, and often a lack of authority, often causing conflicts of interest when doctors/managers attempt to do their job (Naamati-Schneider, 2022).

Unclear job descriptions and undefined on-the-job authority are also associated with a decreased sense of accountability, a lack of transparency, and a lack of understanding of the extent of individual responsibility. These factors create instability and constitute a situation that is liable to generate medical and managerial problems (Figueroa et al., 2019; Krijgsheld et al., 2022).

In addition, healthcare systems and organizations face internal complexities in human resource management, marked by personal dilemmas and conflicts. These issues are compounded by organizational tensions between managers and medical staff, which further contribute to conflicts and dilemmas within the system. The resulting tension is detrimental to the system and those working within it (Figueroa et al., 2019; Naamati-Schneider et al., 2024a, 2024b).

Altering the healthcare system to focus on patients also has an impact at the micro level. This alteration requires changing the nature and quality of the relationship between patients and healthcare professionals, a relationship previously characterized by a paternalistic approach on the part of the professionals. In the structured, asymmetrical relationship of the past, the healthcare professional possessed the knowledge and authority and therefore made the decisions, while the patient accepted these decisions. The shift to a patient-centered approach has brought about changes in this relationship. The patient environment has changed as well. Consumerism and digital innovations now provide patients free access to sources of information easily available on the Internet. Patients can interact with experts and other patients through a variety of online medical forums and can manage their health services online.

This change in the relationship between the patient and the healthcare professional has forced both sides to adopt different patterns of work and conduct. These changes have resulted in a customer-focused approach to treatment characterized by cooperation between healthcare provider and patients. The process has empowered patients and energized them to play a more active role in their own healthcare. At the same time, healthcare professionals and organizations have been forced to make cultural, organizational, managerial, and personal changes to create trust and teamwork that will improve patients' responses and enhance their treatment (Prag et al., 2017). Making these changes requires changing the focus, developing teamwork skills, and adopting a new perspective in setting goals. As an integral part of these changes, healthcare personnel must develop interpersonal communication skills and the ability to provide information and guidance (Aka Zohar, 2019). Figure 2.1 illustrates the changing ecosystem of the healthcare industry relative to the three system levels and the stressors affecting the system and its workforce.

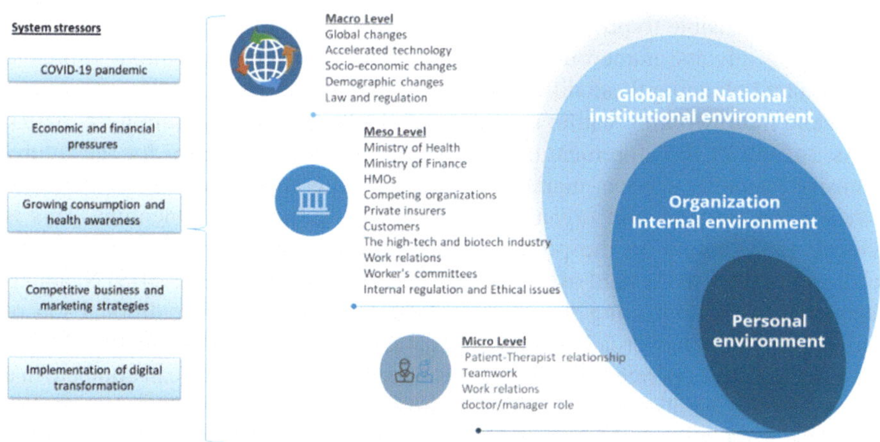

Fig. 2.1 The changing ecosystem of the healthcare industry

Implementing these changes throughout the system requires significant adaptation and change on all three levels. These changes demand cooperation, effective communication, and inter- and intra-organizational collaboration in working toward a common goal. Successfully implementing these changes requires developing leadership skills at all levels so as to assimilate the change and transform it into a guiding principle in the development healthcare professionals (Naamati-Schneider, 2020). Moreover, these processes of change point to the growing need for programs and content suitable to twenty-first century healthcare systems and organizations that must deal with these far-reaching changes on a daily basis.

The Need for Skilled Medical Management

The changes in the healthcare system and its environment are expected to continue and even gather momentum. The prediction is that the demand for healthcare services and products will continue to grow without any additional budgetary allotment for healthcare, thus widening the gap between demand and what healthcare services can offer (WHO, 2019). Future worsening of this situation will only highlight and place renewed emphasis on these issues, as well as on the need to develop and adopt changes in the system and its management (Counte et al., 2019). At the same time, in recent years new technologies for distance treatment and diagnosis as well as blockchain technology, applications and artificial intelligence have been incorporated into the healthcare system. These technologies will continue to shape the digital transformation in the near and far future (Davenport & Kalakota, 2019; Gupta et al., 2019; Siyal et al., 2019; Wang & Preininger, 2019).

Indeed, these new technologies will facilitate changes in treatment and hospitalization services that will place emphasis on improving patients' experiences and community and home hospitalization (Counte et al., 2019). These ongoing changes will make it possible to provide more efficient and higher quality services. Nevertheless, they involve numerous difficulties and if implemented without sufficient direction and planning these difficulties are liable to exacerbate for the system as a whole and those working within it (Bitkina et al., 2020; Wang & Preininger, 2019).

As a result of the aforementioned processes and in preparation for the future, extensive business, service, marketing-oriented and competition-oriented changes in healthcare systems and organization have been gathering momentum. This is evident, for example, in the proliferation of new academic study programs and academic degrees in the field of medical management (Counte et al., 2019; Naamati-Schneider, 2020), reflecting the current understanding that the traditional job of medical providers has broadened beyond patient diagnosis and treatment. Healthcare systems must operate as profitable business organizations that can compete in a free market with public and private healthcare organizations and with various bodies within the same system. Moreover, today's globalization and information accessibility have eliminated geographical catchment areas and encouraged the opening of the global market (Naamati-Schneider, 2021; Naamati-Schneider& Zaks, 2022).

Consequently, health management has become an existential necessity for healthcare systems at all levels. This includes the role of hybrid professional managers who combine professional expertise in a specific health-related field, such as medicine, nursing, or allied health professions, with managerial skills and responsibilities or designated healthcare managers, these professionals play a crucial role in the healthcare sector. Understanding the complex nature of business management at all levels is an integral part of managing health organizations. Indeed, health management includes determining health policies, setting general holistic strategy, organizational management, planning, budgeting, establishing an organizational culture, managing human resources and managing customer services (Raftery et al., 2022).

Discussion

Despite the above, most educational programs in the field of healthcare system management still focus on improving values and not necessarily on issues of service, management quality, leadership or effective adaptation to environmental changes (Counte et al., 2019).

Clearly, managers in the field of healthcare must be trained to adapt to the changes and complexities of the system described here. In 2015 an international consortium of healthcare system directors met to discuss the issue of healthcare management professionalization (Global Consortium for Healthcare Management Professionalization, 2015). The consortium issued a document describing the changes in the field and the need for a precise definition of management in the area of healthcare. The document cited specific objectives and skills needed to develop healthcare management professionals who are in tune with the changing environment. The main problems discussed focused on the central needs of medical management, the issue of gaining recognition for this field, and the importance of guidance, training, and education to attain specific abilities and skills. The consortium issued an urgent call for governments and healthcare communities to recognize that performance and improvement in the healthcare field are highly dependent on the existence and quality of professional management of healthcare organizations. It also urged them to nurture abilities toward developing ethical, just, and egalitarian behavior among medical managers and to provide them with leadership and education to transform them into lifelong learners of these skills (Global Consortium for Healthcare Management Professionalization, 2015; Hahn & Gil Lapetra, 2019).

Consequently, researchers worldwide (Alt et al., 2023; Counte et al., 2019; Dolev et al., 2021; Raftery et al., 2022) have called for broadening the scope of medical education and management programs in an effort to deal with these problems and changes in the healthcare system, while specifically referring to the need for healthcare system personnel to adapt to these changes. Education in the field of medical management is required for planning, executing, and evaluating financial plans in order to improve effectiveness and quality. Managers and medical professionals must be trained to adapt to the market demands in this field. Proper training includes identifying the entire range of necessary qualifications and specific skills that will contribute to leadership and effective management of healthcare systems and organizations. This training will benefit healthcare systems, organizations, and staff to make them as sustainable as possible during current processes of changes as well as the unknown changes in the future (Counte et al., 2019; Raftery et al., 2022).

Training should be broad and comprehensive and cover a range of competencies and skills that will enable people to adapt to these processes and manage current changes and those expected in the near and distant future. These twenty-first century skills are divided into three levels—cognitive, intrapersonal, and interpersonal (National Research Council, 2012; Rios et al., 2020)—and among other things include problem-solving, argumentation, creativity, collaboration, literacy, self-regulation, ethical judgment and leadership skills.

This book focuses on developing these competencies and skills among health system managers through competency-based learning methods. It seeks to address the gaps in the existing curriculum as well as the needs of different health systems in coping with current processes of change and adaptation.

References

Aka Zohar, A. (2019). *Eichut be-mifgash metapel metupal: Tfisa hadasha* [Quality in the encounter between clinician and patient: A new approach]. In S. Shafran-Sigal, Y. Shemer, & Y. Weiss (Eds.), *Mifgashim be'olam habriut* [*Encounters in the world of health*] (pp. 235–272). Akademon. (Hebrew)

Alt, D., Naamati-Schneider, L., & Weishut, D. J. (2023). Competency-based learning and formative assessment feedback as precursors of college students' soft skills acquisition. *Studies in Higher Education*, 1–17. https://doi.org/10.1080/03075079.2023.2217203

Argenziano, M., Fischkoff, K., & Smith, C. R. (2020). Surgery scheduling in a crisis. *New England Journal of Medicine*. https://doi.org/10.1056/NEJMc2017424

Arora, S., Ashrafian, H., Davis, R., Athanasiou, T., Darzi, A., & Sevdalis, N. (2010). Emotional intelligence in medicine: a systematic review through the context of the ACGME competencies. *Medical education, 44*(8), 749–764.

Azzolini, E., Ricciardi, W., & Gray, M. (2018). Healthcare organizational performance: Why changing the culture really matters. *Commentary. Ann Ist Super Sanita, 54*(1), 6–8. https://doi.org/10.4415/ANN_18_01_03. PMID: 29616667.

Bar, A. (2020, July 4). The positive side of the Coronavirus—A digital leap forward: People have discovered the internet's capabilities. https://www.bizportal.co.il/general/news/article/781921 (Hebrew)

Bin-Nun, G. (2019). Equality, equitability, and everything in between. The case of the health system in Israel. In S. Shafran & Y. Weiss (Eds.), *Encounters in the world of health* (pp. 328–338). Magnes (Hebrew)

Bitkina, O. V., Kim, H. K., & Park, J. (2020). Usability and user experience of medical devices: An overview of the current state, analysis methodologies, and future challenges. *International Journal of Industrial Ergonomics, 76*, 102932. https://doi.org/10.1016/j.ergon.2020.102932

Bozorgmehr, K., Saint, V., Kaasch, A., Stuckler, D., & Kentikelenis, A. (2020). COVID and the convergence of three crises in Europe. *The Lancet Public Health, 5*(5), e247–e248.https://doi.org/10.1016/s2468-2667(20)30078-5

Bruno, A., Dell'Aversana, G., & Zunino, A. (2017). Customer orientation and leadership in the health service sector: the role of workplace social support. *Frontiers in Psychology, 8*, 1920. https://doi.org/10.3389/fpsyg.2017.01920

Cernega, A., Nicolescu, D. N., Meleşcanu Imre, M., Ripszky Totan, A., Arsene, A. L., Şerban, R. S., Perpelea AC, Nedea MI, & Piţuru, S. M. (2024). Volatility, Uncertainty, Complexity, and Ambiguity (VUCA) n Healthcare. In *Healthcare, 12*(7), 773. https://doi.org/10.3390/healthcare12070773

Counte, M. A., Howard, S. W., Chang, L., & Aaronson, W. (2019). Global advances in value-based payment and their implications for global health management education, development, and practice. *Frontiers in Public Health, 6*, 379. https://doi.org/10.3389/fpubh.2018.00379

Davenport, T., & Kalakota, R. (2019). The potential for artificial intelligence in healthcare. *Future Healthcare Journal, 6*(2), 94. https://doi.org/10.7861/futurehosp.6-2-94

Dolev, N., Naamati-Schneider, L., & Meirovich, A. (2021). Making soft skills a part of the curriculum of healthcare studies. In *Medical Education for the 21st Century*. IntechOpen.

Figueroa, C. A., Harrison, R., Chauhan, A., & Meyer, L. (2019). Priorities and challenges for health leadership and workforce management globally: A rapid review. *BMC Health Services Research, 19*(1), 1–11. https://doi.org/10.1186/s12913-019-4080-7

Ginter, P. M., Duncan, W. J., & Swayne, L. E. (2018). *The strategic management of health care organisations*. Wiley.

Global Consortium for Healthcare Management Professionalization. (2015). *International hospital federation. Leadership competencies for healthcare services managers*. https://www.ihf-fih.org/

Global Observatory for eHealth. (2022). Directory of eHealth policies. *World Health Organisation*. http://www.who.int/goe/policies/en/

Gupta, R., Tanwar, S., Tyagi, S., & Kumar, N. (2019). Tactile-internet-based telesurgery system for healthcare 4.0: An architecture, research challenges, and future directions. *IEEE Network, 33*(6), 22–29. https://doi.org/10.1109/MNET.001.1900063

Hahn, C. A., & Gil Lapetra, M. (2019). Development and use of the leadership competencies for healthcare services managers assessment. *Frontiers in Public Health, 7*, 34. https://doi.org/10.3389/fpubh.2019.00034

Hall, W., Williams, I., Smith, N., Gold, M., Coast, J., Kapiriri, L., Danis, M., & Mitton, C. (2018). Past, present and future challenges in health care priority setting: Findings from an international expert survey. *Journal of Health Organization and Management, 32*, 444–462. https://doi.org/10.1108/JHOM-01-2018-0005

Iliffe, S., & Manthorpe, J. (2020). Medical consumerism and the modern patient: Successful ageing, self-management and the 'fantastic prosumer.' *Journal of the Royal Society of Medicine, 113*(9), 339–345.

Keasberry, J., Scott, I. A., Sullivan, C., Staib, A., & Ashby, R. (2017). Going digital: A narrative overview of the clinical and organisational impacts of eHealth technologies in hospital practice. *Australian Health Review, 41*(6), 646–664. https://doi.org/10.1071/AH16233

Kraus, S., Schiavone, F., Pluzhnikova, A., & Invernizzi, A. C. (2021). Digital transformation in healthcare: Analyzing the current state-of-research. *Journal of Business Research, 123*, 557–567. https://doi.org/10.1016/j.jbusres.2020.10.030

Krijgsheld, M., Tummers, L. G. & Scheepers, F. E. (2022). Job performance in healthcare: a systematic review. *BMC Health Services Research* 22, 149. https://doi.org/10.1186/s12913-021-07357-5

Marques, I. C. P., & Ferreira, J. J. M. (2020). Digital transformation in the area of health: Systematic review of 45 years of evolution. *Health and Technology, 10*(3), 575–586. https://doi.org/10.1007/s12553-019-00402-8

Mercer, D., Haddon, A., & Loughlin, C. (2018). Leading on the edge: The nature of paramedic leadership at the front line of care. *Health Care Management Review, 43*(1), 12–20. https://doi.org/10.1097/HMR.0000000000000125

Naamati Schneider, L. (2020). Strategic management as an adaptation to changes in the ecosystems of public hospitals in Israel. *Israel Journal of Health Policy Research, 9*, 65. https://doi.org/10.1186/s13584-020-00424-y

Naamati Schneider, L. (2021). Public-private: Unequal competition: Israeli public hospitals versus the private healthcare system following government reforms. *International Journal of Organisational Analysis*. https://doi.org/10.1108/IJOA-06-2020-2237

Naamati-Schneider, L. (2022). Intraorganisation conflicts of interest in hospitals adapting to a changing ecosystem. *Journal of Health Organisation and Management*. https://doi.org/10.1108/jhom-09-2021-0325

Naamati-Schneider, L. (2023). The effect of digitalization on service orientation and service perception among Israeli healthcare professionals: A qualitative study. *Digital Health, 9*, https://doi.org/10.1177/20552076231191892

Naamati-Schneider, L., Arazi-Fadlon, M., & Daphna-Tekoah, S. (2024a). Strategic technological processes in hospitals: Conflicts and personal experiences of healthcare teams. *Nursing Ethics. 0*(0). https://doi.org/10.1177/09697330241252876

Naamati-Schneider, L., Arazi-Fadlon, M. & Daphna-Tekoah, S. (2024b). Navigating moral and ethical dilemmas and conflict in strategic technological processes within healthcare organizations. *Digital Health.*

Naamati-Schneider, L., Salvatore, F. P. (2023). Sustainability for Healthcare Organisations and Systems: Cultivating Strategy and Governance Processes for a Better Future. In: Vrontis, D., Thrassou, A., Efthymiou, L., Weber, Y., Shams, S.M.R., Tsoukatos, E. (Eds.), *Business for sustainability,* Volume I. pp.227–249. Palgrave Studies in Cross-disciplinary Business Research, In Association with EuroMed Academy of Business. Palgrave Macmillan, Cham. https://doi.org/10.1007/978-3-031-37361-9_11

Naamati-Schneider, L., & Zaks, O. (2022). Public hospitals in crisis: Managerial and strategic adaptation. In D. Vrontis, A. Thrassou, Y. Weber, S. M. R. Shams, E. Tsoukatos, & L. Efthymiou (Eds.), *Business under crisis: Volume II* (pp. 43–64). Palgrave Macmillan. https://doi.org/10.1007/978-3-030-76575-0_3

National Research Council. (2012). *Education for life and work: Developing transferable knowledge and skills in the 21st century.* National Academies Press.

Nilsen, P., Seing, I., Ericsson, C., et al. (2020). Characteristics of successful changes in health care organizations: An interview study with physicians, registered nurses and assistant nurses. *BMC Health Services Research, 20*, 147. https://doi.org/10.1186/s12913-020-4999-8

OECD. (2020). *Organisation for economic cooperation and development global health spending data.* Retrieved from https://data.oecd.org/healthres/health-spending.htm.

Otter, K. (2019). Developing leadership: Innovation, adaptability and integration in large-scale health care organizations. *Experten führen: Modelle, Ideen und Praktiken für die Organisations- und Führungsentwicklung*, 179-192. https://doi.org/10.1007/978-3-658-23028-9_10

Papanicolas, I., Woskie, L. R., & Jha, A. K. (2018). Health care spending in the united states and other high-income countries. *JAMA, 319*(10), 1024–1039. https://doi.org/10.1001/jama.2018.1150

Potluri, R. M., & Johnson, S. (2023). Healthcare Consumerism and Implications for Care Delivery. In *Medical Entrepreneurship: Trends and Prospects in the Digital Age* (pp. 199–211). Springer.

Präg, P., Wittek, R., & Mills, M. C. (2017). The educational gradient in self-rated health in Europe: Does the doctor–patient relationship make a difference? *Acta Sociologica, 60*(4), 325–341. https://doi.org/10.1177/0001699316670715

Raftery, C., Sassenberg, A. M., & Bamford-Wade, A. (2022). Business acumen for nursing leaders: An exploratory qualitative study. *Journal of Nursing Management*. https://doi-org.mgs.hac.ac.il/10.1111/jonm.13672

Reijula, J., Reijula, E., & Reijula, K. (2016). Healthcare management challenges in two university hospitals. *International Journal of Healthcare Technology and Management, 15*(4), 308–325. https://doi.org/10.1504/IJHTM.2016.084129

Reis, S. (2019). The doctor in the digital age competencies needed and a road map for their achievement [review]. *Harefuah. 158*(10), 648–653) Hebrew)

Reis, S., Visser, A., & Frankel, R. (2013). Health information and communication technology in healthcare communication: The good, the bad, and the transformative. *Patient Education and Counseling, 93*(3), 359–362. https://doi.org/10.1016/j.pec.2013.10.007

Ricciardi, W., Pita Barros, P., Bourek, A., Brouwer, W., Kelsey, T., & Lehtonen, L. (2019). How to govern the digital transformation of health services. *European Journal of Public Health, 29*, 7–12. https://doi.org/10.1093/eurpub/ckz165

Rios, J. A., Ling, G., Pugh, R., Becker, D., & Bacall, A. (2020). Identifying critical 21st-century skills for workplace success: A content analysis of job advertisements. *Educational Researcher, 49*(2), 80–89. https://doi.org/10.3102/0013189X19890600

Ron, R., & Weiss, R. (2020). The ramifications of reducing elective activity in hospitals during the Coronavirus crisis: Insights and conclusions. *Harefua, 159*(7), 475–476. (Hebrew).

Schwab, K. (2017). *The fourth industrial revolution*. Currency.

Siyal, A. A., Junejo, A. Z., Zawish, M., Ahmed, K., Khalil, A., & Soursou, G. (2019). Applications of blockchain technology in medicine and healthcare: Challenges and future perspectives. *Cryptography, 3*(1), 3. https://doi.org/10.3390/cryptography3010003

Thorpe, K. E., Ogden, L. L., & Galactionova, K. (2010). Chronic conditions account for rise in Medicare spending from 1987 to 2006. *Health Affairs, 29*(4), 718–724.

Tjahjono, B., Esplugues, C., Ares, E., & Pelaez, G. (2017). What does industry 4.0 mean to supply chain? *Procedia Manufacturing, 13*, 1175–1182. https://doi.org/10.1016/j.promfg.2017.09.191

Torugsa, N. A., O'Donohue, W., & Hecker, R. (2012). Capabilities, proactive CSR and financial performance in SMEs: Empirical evidence from an Australian manufacturing industry sector. *Journal of Business Ethics, 109*, 483–500.

Tung, W., Liang, A. R. D., & Chen, S. C. (2014). The influence of service orientation and interaction orientation on consumer identification. *The Service Industries Journal, 34*(5), 439–454. https://doi.org/10.1080/02642069.2014.871533

United Nations. (2016). Sustainable development. *Department of Economic and Social Affairs*. https://www.un.org/sustainabledevelopment/sustainable-development-goals/

Wang, F., & Preininger, A. (2019). AI in health: State of the art, challenges, and future directions. *Yearbook of Medical Informatics, 28*(01), 16–26. https://doi.org/10.1055/s-0039-1677908

WHO. (2019). *World Health Organisation: Universal health coverage*. Retrieved from https://www.who.int/news-room/fact-sheets/detail/universal-health-coverage-(uhc). June 2022.

World Economic Forum. (2015). *New vision for education: Unlocking the potential of technology*. World Economic Forum.

Worley, C. G., & Jules, C. (2020). COVID-19's uncomfortable revelations about agile and sustainable organizations in a VUCA world. *The Journal of Applied Behavioral Science, 56*(3), 279–283. https://doi.org/10.1177/0021886320936263

Zangrandi A., Fanelli S., Donelli C. C., & Elefanti M. (2020). *Crisis managment: la gestione di un ospedale durante una pandemia*. EGEA.

Chapter 3
Competency-Based Learning and Real-World Performance in Health Management Professions

Abstract In today's rapidly evolving healthcare landscape, equipping students with 21st-century skills (21CS) is more crucial than ever. Drawing upon the 21CS taxonomy proposed by the National Research Council and other contemporary classifications, this chapter examines how students can effectively acquire these essential skills. Emphasizing competency-based learning approaches that focus on measurable outcomes, it explores the impact on students' cognitive, intra-personal, and inter-personal 21CS. By providing a comprehensive definition of 21CS and showcasing their application within health management curricula, the chapter highlights their growing importance in academia and the job market.

Introduction

twenty-first century skills (21CS) are of critical importance to health managers in striving to adapt to today's rapidly changing conditions. These skills include the ability to solve complex problems, collaborate and communicate effectively with others, and self-regulate learning processes (Tindowen et al., 2017). Yet despite worldwide acknowledgment of their importance, very few educational systems have integrated these skills into their framework. Hence, although these skills have been deemed important in coping effectively with changes, higher education systems have failed to establish a comprehensive instructional framework to help design competency-based learning approaches, thus falling short when it comes to nurturing students' 21CS (Vista, 2020).

The challenge of incorporating twenty-first century skills is the focus of this chapter. Drawing on the 21CS taxonomy of the National Research Council (2012) and on contemporary classifications associated with health management (American College of Healthcare Executives, 2022), the chapter outlines the type of learning experiences that may help students acquire 21CS. More specifically, it focuses on competency-based learning environments employed by faculty members. The traditional teaching paradigm centered primarily on recitation and memorization techniques. Through the use of interactive methods, competency-based learning has

L. Naamati-Schneider and D. Alt, *Technology and Competency-Oriented Learning*,
https://doi.org/10.1007/978-981-97-5771-8_3

begun to shift this paradigm toward constructivist approaches aimed at enhancing students' skills (European Commission, 2018). The chapter discusses the impact of these settings on students' perceived cognitive, intrapersonal, and interpersonal 21CS. In doing so, it provides valuable insights into the development of competency-based learning methods and specific learning and instructional activities that may enhance the 21CS of students in higher education. The chapter provides a comprehensive definition of 21CS and describes their increasing importance as outlined in the literature and reflected on the job market. Then, it defines the concept of competency-based learning. Finally, it shows how competency-based learning methods have been used and researched in the context of health management curricula.

21st Century Skills

Despite the many studies stressing the importance of 21CS, there is very little consensus regarding how to define these skills, whether they are malleable, how they can be enhanced, and how they should be measured. Researchers such as Redecker et al. (2011) and others have identified three general categories of 21CS: (1) personal skills (e.g., initiative, resilience, and creativity); (2) social skills (e.g., team, networking, empathy, and compassion); and (3) learning skills (e.g., organizational and metacognitive skills). Other research initiatives (e.g., Partnership for 21st Century Skills, 2014) have classified 21CS into life and career skills; learning and innovation skills (including critical thinking, communication, collaboration, and creativity); and information media and technology skills. Binkley et al. (2012) proposed classifying 21CS into three categories: ways of thinking, ways of working, and ways of living in the world. The Organization for Economic Cooperation and Development (OECD) proposed a three-dimensional framework consisting of information, communication and ethics, and social impact. It focuses on skills in information literacy, data literacy, and digital content creation; effective digital communication, ethical technology use, and cultural awareness; and promoting digital citizenship, social responsibility, and innovation. This comprehensive approach ensures individuals are equipped with the necessary skills to navigate, contribute to, and responsibly engage with the digital world, addressing both technical abilities and the ethical, social, and cultural implications of digital technology.

This chapter centers on the taxonomy proposed by the National Research Council (2012), which is quite detailed and used extensively in numerous studies and documents (Nehring et al., 2019; Oliveri & Mislevy, 2019; Rios et al., 2020). This taxonomy (Table 3.1) was specifically developed for the US National Academy of Sciences and later adopted in the report of the US Department of Education (Shectman et al., 2013). Drawing on previous literature such as Bloom's (1956) cognitive and affective taxonomies and Carroll's (1993) taxonomy of cognitive abilities, this classification scheme includes three core competence domains—cognitive, intrapersonal, and interpersonal—that are associated with eight "clusters" of 21CS competencies: (1) Cognitive Processes and Strategies (CPS); (2) Knowledge; (3)

Creativity; (4) Intellectual Openness; (5) Work Ethic/Conscientiousness; (6) Positive Core Self-Evaluation; (7) Teamwork and Collaboration; and (8) Leadership.

In the context of health management, the American College of Healthcare Executives report (2022) outlined a more specific sets of skills covered by the above detailed taxonomy. The report further suggested an updated assessment tool (Healthcare Executive Competencies Assessment Tool) that healthcare leaders can use in assessing their expertise in critical areas of healthcare management. The competencies were derived from job analysis surveys of healthcare leaders across various management and administration disciplines and are categorized into five domains (p. 3):

Table 3.1 Twenty-first century competency clusters

Competency type	Cluster	Terms used for 21st century skills
Cognitive	Cognitive processes and strategies	Critical thinking; problem solving; analysis; reasoning/argumentation; interpretation; decision-making; adaptive learning; executive function
	Knowledge	Information literacy (research using evidence and recognizing bias in sources); information and communications technology literacy; oral and written communication; active listening
	Creativity	Creativity, innovation
Intrapersonal	Intellectual openness	Flexibility; adaptability; artistic and cultural appreciation; personal and social responsibility (including cultural awareness and competence); appreciation of diversity; adaptability; continuous learning; intellectual interest and curiosity
	Work ethic/ conscientiousness	Initiative; self-direction; responsibility; perseverance; productivity; grit; Type 1 self-regulation (metacognitive skills; including forethought, performance, and self-reflection); professionalism/ethics; integrity; citizenship; career orientation
	Positive core self-evaluation	Type 2 self-regulation (self-monitoring; self-evaluation; self-reinforcement); physical and psychological health
Interpersonal	Teamwork and collaboration	Communication; collaboration; teamwork; cooperation; coordination; interpersonal skills; empathy/perspective taking; trust; service orientation; conflict resolution; negotiation
	Leadership	Leadership; responsibility; assertive communication; self-presentation; social influence with others

Source National Research Council (2012)

1. Communication and Relationship Management: The ability to communicate clearly and concisely with internal and external customers, establish and maintain relationships, and facilitate constructive interactions with individuals and groups.
2. Leadership: The ability to inspire individual and organizational excellence, create a shared vision, and successfully manage change to attain the organization's strategic ends and successful performance. Leadership intersects with each of the other four domains.
3. Professionalism: The ability to align personal and organizational conduct with ethical and professional standards, including responsibility to the patient and the community, a service orientation, and a commitment to lifelong learning and improvement.
4. Knowledge of the Healthcare Environment: Understanding the healthcare system and the environment in which healthcare managers and providers operate.
5. Business Skills and Knowledge: The ability to apply business principles, including systems thinking, to the healthcare environment.

Note that although researchers tend to use the terms twenty-first century "skills" and twenty-first century "competencies" interchangeably, the National Research Council (2012, p. 3) has made a clear distinction between these concepts:

> In contrast to a view of 21st Century Skills as general skills that can be applied to a range of different tasks in various ... contexts, the committee views 21st Century Skills as dimensions of expertise that are specific to—and intertwined with—knowledge within a particular domain of content and performance. To reflect our view that skills and knowledge are intertwined, we use the term 'competencies' rather than 'skills'.

In this chapter we use the term "21st century competencies" when referring to the National Research Council's scheme, whereas in discussions concerning other studies we adhere to the more frequently used term—"21st-century skills" (21CS).

The following section is organized according to the three domains suggested by the National Research Council (2012) taxonomy. The discussion also refers to competencies suggested by contemporary classifications such as the ACHE Healthcare Executive 2022 Competencies Assessment Tool (American College of Healthcare Executives, 2022).

Cognitive Competencies

The first domain introduced by the National Research Council (2012) taxonomy refers to a core cognitive competency that includes cognitive processes and strategies, knowledge, and creativity. This domain incorporates competencies such as problem-solving, exercising sound reasoning and critical thinking, generating new ideas and integrating existing ideas in a real-world setting, and information and digital literacy (van Laar et al., 2020). Finding innovative solutions to poorly structured problems requires a certain degree of creativity. Creativity is a form of problem-solving that employs divergent thinking and explores multiple possible solutions to generate ideas. Sawyer (2021) showed how creative work on the part of students is socially constructed and suggested practices for scaffolding students toward mastering a dialogue of creativity. For example, instead of providing specific answers to questions, professors should encourage their students "to explore possibilities and to look for emergence from a continuing dialogue" and "resolve the ambiguity through exploration" (p. 25).

Problem-based learning appears to have potential in fostering student creativity and in influencing several measures of creative thinking, among them fluency and originality in problem-solving, divergent thinking and flexibility, and novel and creative problem-solving. Researchers such as Alt and Raichel (2020) found an association between current global changes and the need for creativity. They recognized this association as a key to success in a continuously changing and challenging world that requires prompt adaptation to new situations. Therefore, enhancing these competencies should become a fundamental goal of higher education in preparing students for future careers.

In the context of healthcare management, the American College of Healthcare Executives report (2022) contends that two competencies can be linked to this cognitive facet: knowledge of the healthcare environment and business skills and knowledge. For example, health and healthcare environment competencies include the ability to demonstrate an understanding of system structure, funding mechanisms, and the organizational structure of healthcare services. Moreover, these competencies entail assessing organizational performance as part of the health system/healthcare services; demonstrating the ability to optimize the healthcare workforce around local critical workforce issues; recognizing and promoting the perspectives of patients and their families/caregivers in the delivery of care; using vital statistics and core health indicators to guide decision-making; and recognizing the local implications of global health events to understand global interconnectivity and its impact on population health conditions.

The business skills and knowledge competencies required in this context include the ability to demonstrate knowledge of basic business practices and seek information from a variety of sources to support organizational performance; effective use of key accounting principles and financial management tools; planning, organizing, executing and monitoring organizational resources; effectively managing departmental human resource processes; demonstrating knowledge of governmental, regulatory, professional and accreditation agencies and of the role of leadership within the governmental structure; planning for business continuity in the face of potential disasters that can disrupt service delivery; ensuring that applicable privacy and security requirements are upheld; being able to develop and implement quality assurance, satisfaction, and patient safety programs.

Intrapersonal Competencies

The intrapersonal domain involves three sets of competencies: intellectual openness, work ethic, and positive self-evaluation. Of these, self-regulation is perceived as a core ability (National Research Council, 2012). Self-regulation refers to students' ability to understand and control their learning (Alt & Naamati-Schneider, 2021b; Schunk & Zimmerman, 1994) to the point of becoming metacognitively, motivationally, and behaviorally active in their own learning processes. Self-regulated learners metacognitively control and regulate skills needed for planning, monitoring, and modifying cognition. They are able to use cognitive strategies to pursue academic goals and strategies that empower them to self-monitor their own learning (Zimmerman & Moylan, 2009). These learners can monitor their own progress while working on a task and can adjust strategies to foster success. Self-regulated students frequently raise questions, take notes, and manage their resources in ways that help them control their learning. Self-regulated learning strategies are essential to prepare students for lifelong learning and are deemed an important capacity for transferring skills and knowledge across domains and settings (Schuster et al., 2020).

In the context of healthcare management, the American College of Healthcare Executives report (2022) suggests that the following competencies are linked to this facet: self-awareness of one's own assumptions, values, strengths, and limitations and the ability to demonstrate reflective leadership by using self-assessment and feedback from others; ethical conduct and social consciousness, for example by using established ethical structures to resolve ethical issues and demonstrating high ethical conduct; and professional development and lifelong learning through a demonstrated commitment to self-development that incorporates continuing education, networking, reflection and personal improvement.

Interpersonal Competencies

The interpersonal domain includes competencies such as effectively communicating multiple types of information, interpreting messages across multiple forms of audiences, collaborating with diverse teams, and managing conflicts, together with presenting ideas clearly and effectively and demonstrating integrity and ethical behavior (Markle et al., 2013). Borge and White (2016) emphasized the importance of honing students' ability toward understanding and regulating collaborative interactions through instructional frameworks. Yet despite the importance of these competencies in preparing the future generation to confront the challenges of real-life situations, educational institutions worldwide tend to center more on the cognitive aspects of learning while neglecting its socio-metacognitive aspects (Alt & Raichel, 2021). To meet the challenges of globalization, institutions of higher learning must focus on fundamental soft skills that are considered critical components of success in the workplace, including communication, teamwork, collaboration, and leadership skills. Through content analysis of 142,000 online job advertisements, Rios et al. (2020) empirically investigated which 21CS are essential for students in higher education to make the transition to the workforce. Their findings indicate that employers gave precedence to oral and written communication, collaboration, and problem-solving skills over other skills such as social responsibility.

The International Hospital Federation (2015) emphasized leadership as a core competency needed for healthcare managers and divided leadership into four sub-categories (p. 6). The first sub-category, *Leadership Skills and Behavior*, incorporated the following: articulating and communicating the organization's mission, objectives and priorities to internal and external entities; incorporating management techniques and theories into leadership activities; analyzing problems, promoting solutions and encouraging decision making. The second sub-category, *Engaging Culture and Environment*, entailed creating an organizational climate built on mutual trust, transparency and a focus on service improvement that encourages teamwork and supports diversity; encouraging a high level of commitment from employees by establishing and communicating a compelling organizational vision and goals; and holding self and others accountable for surpassing organizational goals. The third sub-category, *Leading Change*, included promoting ongoing learning and improvement in the organization, responding to the need for change, and leading the change process. The fourth sub-category, *Driving Innovation*, referred to diverse thinking to support innovation, creativity, and improvement.

Based on the American College of Healthcare Executives report (2022), several healthcare management competencies can be linked to interpersonal competencies: relationship management—demonstrating effective interpersonal relationships and collaborative techniques for engaging and working with stakeholders; communication skills and engagement, comprising the ability to exercise cultural sensitivity in internal and external communication and to demonstrate strong listening and communication skills; and facilitation and negotiation, including the ability to manage conflict through mediation and build and participate in effective multidisciplinary teams.

Twenty-first century competencies are deemed important for professionalizing healthcare management and producing highly competent managers. Yet despite being considered important skills, "education systems are only just beginning to formalize the frameworks for the teaching and learning of these skills" (Vista, 2020, p. 1). The following section illustrates how higher education programs can enhance students' cognitive, intrapersonal, and interpersonal competencies by embracing the pedagogical approach of competency-based learning.

Soft Skills: Intrapersonal and Interpersonal Competencies

Soft skills involve intrapersonal and interpersonal competencies essential for optimal functioning in general, and particularly in contemporary work environments (Succi & Canovi, 2020). Several models have been proposed to define and classify soft skills, among them life skills (Ammani & Chitra, 2020); twenty-first century skills (Lepeley et al., 2021), key competencies for a successful life, and lifelong learning (OECD, 2012). Soft skills require an optimal combination of emotion and thought and include the ability to identify, understand, use, and manage feelings (Khaouja et al., 2019).

Soft skills are used in a host of professions (Barrera-Osorio et al., 2020). In clinical and medical fields, including medical management, such skills are considered as prerequisites and core competencies. In the context of healthcare, skills such as effective communication, teamwork, time management, and leadership are an essential part of the medical team's socio-organizational work environment (Bos–van den Hoek et al., 2019). Thus, for example, communication skills are an integral part of what healthcare professionals do every day because they need to communicate with patients, relatives, colleagues, and administrative staff (Yao et al., 2021). Soft skills have been found to be correlated with medical leadership, effective functioning under pressure, positive interpersonal communication, and good teamwork (Tripathy, 2020); with improved patient-therapist relationships, providing patients with empathic treatment, and improved patient satisfaction and trust (Dimitrov & Vazova, 2020); and with greater accuracy in medical diagnosis and subsequently in medical treatment, a reduction in patients' situational anxiety, and an increase in patients' willingness to undergo treatment (Back et al., 2020).

Competency-Based Learning

The traditional teaching paradigm focuses primarily on rote memorization of factual knowledge. Competency-based learning shifts this paradigm toward constructivist approaches aimed at enhancing students' skills and sense of agency and thus turning them into more active individuals (European Commission, 2018). According to learner-centered environment approaches, learning occurs during active participation in inquiry practices (Alt & Raichel, 2021). Competency-based learning approaches encourage teachers to place students in authentic tasks and pay attention to students' views on task relevance. Educators in such environments provide multiple representations of the content and foster dialogue, thereby helping learners deal with how to acquire knowledge within rapid processes of change. Inquiry practices are utilized to support the development of critical thinking as they facilitate open inquiry based on authentic and loosely structured problems. Learners are required to draw on new and prior knowledge, skills, and approaches when providing solutions and must design new paths toward solving problems while generating new knowledge (European Commission, 2018).

Students engaged in competency-based learning approaches are provided with opportunities to actively participate in self-regulated learning processes. (Alt & Naamati-Schneider, 2021b). They are provided with scaffolding while learning and encouraged to reflect on their own learning processes. In competency-based learning, the teacher is not considered to be a "knowledge authority". Instead, a variety of multidimensional learning methods and content are employed to scaffold each learner's needs and interests.

Competency-based learning approaches also highlight the social and collaborative nature of learning. Learning is often organized into groups in which students are given opportunities to collaborate and learn together. In addition to developing knowledge and skills, students develop their attitudes toward others, often by means of social construction (European Commission, 2018).

Previous research showed how such approaches may positively affect competence development and suggested specific activities to promote the construction of 21CS that are applicable to any subject area (Alt & Raichel, 2018). To develop 21CS, learners must play an active and equal role in constructing their learning, for example by designing participatory learning activities in which learners can be involved in decision-making regarding their learning progression and develop a sense of autonomy and agency through self-reflection. Safe learning environments are required to support competence development. For example, game-based learning environments (Kahila et al., 2020) have been proven effective in promoting emotional and social skills as they offer a safe environment for confronting negative emotions and cooperating with other players to achieve a common goal. Project-based learning enables students to actively explore real-world problems, thereby empowering them as critical thinkers and independent decision-makers who can manage, create, and implement projects while practicing collaborative skills. Project-based activities also enhance students' adaptability, curiosity, sense of responsibility, creativity, technology literacy, problem-solving abilities, self-directed learning, critical thinking, and perseverance (Lai & Guo, 2018).

Intrapersonal skills can be enhanced by generating educational goals that incorporate learner empowerment. This includes developing teaching methods suited to individuals and their abilities that enable students to learn independently and become sensitive to professional-moral aspects. Additionally, these methods should assist students in understanding themselves and recognizing their strengths. To achieve this, the goal-oriented perception of education should shift to a holistic approach that emphasizes the development of the whole individual (Alt & Raichel, 2018). "Whole individuals" are in holistic balance with their emotional, mental, and physical components and with others as well. Educators should reinforce, emphasize, and reveal the qualities of whole individuals by generating activities in which learners must accept commitment, follow their inner beliefs, seek support, use tools to develop consciousness, and cope with difficulties and challenges through opportunities for healing and sharing with others. Proper learning opportunities in which students are empowered and feel safe to express their opinions freely are essential for fostering moral and democratic discussions and values. Furthermore, such opportunities may elicit a heightened sense of self-respect, self-appreciation, self-confidence, self-regulation, and self-efficacy among students.

The use of 21CS has become a well-accepted policy worldwide (Karaca-Atik et al., 2023), reflecting what students need to know and be able to do to flourish in a globalized environment. Nevertheless, Nehring et al. (2019) claim that these skills have not been sufficiently incorporated into educational systems across the globe. One primary reason for not incorporating these skills is the omnipresence of summative assessment methods in many countries, which hinder in-depth learning. These mandated tests are still being used because of problems in "measuring skills beyond the narrow and shallow skill set historically associated with test-based accountability" (p. 10). The fact that people differ considerably with respect to these skills depending upon their circumstances presents another challenge in that assessment necessarily includes significant tradeoffs in foci, methods, and cultural norms (Oliveri & Mislevy, 2019).

21st Century Skills Enhanced by Competency-Based Learning in Health Management Education

Over the past few years, the authors of this book conducted several studies aimed at facilitating the links between effective competency-based learning methods and 21CS among health management students. These methods are discussed in brief in this section and several of them are described at length throughout this volume.

The first cohort of core cognitive competencies includes three clusters: cognitive processes and strategies, knowledge, and creativity. Cognitive processes and strategies are associated with argumentation skills. Alt and Naamati-Schneider (2021a) discussed how the COVID-19 pandemic affected educational systems worldwide, forcing them to shift abruptly from face-to-face to online teaching and learning. They described how a traditional lecture-based activity for undergraduate students in a program for management of health service organizations was transformed into an argumentation-based learning activity using the digital concept mapping technique and how it was deployed in an online format during the COVID-19 lockdown. The students were given the task of solving a poorly structured problem that was connected to the contents of their course on "Assimilation of service quality in health systems". The problem was relevant to their future professional lives. The activity was divided into two phases. In Phase 1, participants were asked to specify five arguments to establish their proposed solution to the problem by using a concept map on a digital platform (*Mindomo*). In Phase 2, they were asked to substantiate their arguments. The participants' impressions of the activity were examined through reflective journals. The qualitative data underwent thematic analysis that entailed searching for themes demonstrating different epistemological positions. Six themes were inductively derived from the students' reflections: (1) transitioning from passive to active learning; (2) generating epistemic change; (3) social perspective-taking; (4) domain-based knowledge; (5) prior knowledge and experience; and (6) online collaboration with other students. To increase the reliability of the recurrent and common themes, students reported specific episodes, thoughts, and feelings. The findings indicated that combining constructivist teaching and learning tools with advanced technology in an online course facilitates the development of lifelong learning capabilities among students in the health management professions.

The knowledge cluster incorporates skills such as information literacy. Alt et al. (2022a) described the implementation of an online Future Problem Solving (FPS) program in the field of health management education. They explored what the program contributed to students' eHealth Literacy identity at two levels of teacher guidance: minimal vs. frequent. A group of 113 Israeli undergraduate students enrolled in a program for management of health service organizations participated in the study. The participating students were divided into two groups—research and control—and FPS was employed in both groups. The 62 students in the research group were given regular weekly guidance that focused on enhancing their eHealth Literacy skills. In the control group, in contrast, the lecturer offered minimal guidance. Data were gathered twice from both groups: pre- and post-program implementation. The findings showed significant differences only for the research group, with levels of eHealth Literacy skills rising between the tests. Moreover, only in the research group did the perception of the FPS program as meaningful contribute to perceived eHealth Literacy skills, whereas the results for the control group were not significant. This study showed that enhancing skills in online educational environments requires frequent and personalized guidance. Faculty members must acknowledge the role of the instructor as a facilitator of learning and must design successful scaffolding strategies to nurture students' lifelong learning skills during distance learning.

In the context of cognitive competencies, the third cluster comprises creativity and innovation. Alt et al. (2022b) emphasized that during the outbreak of the COVID-19 pandemic, online counseling became increasingly necessary to preserve therapeutic processes that were originally conducted in a face-to-face format. Furthermore, the lockdowns exacerbated the need for therapeutic services. Previous studies already pointed out the benefits and effectiveness of online counseling, though these studies claimed a lack of research concerning what therapist characteristics are necessary for online counseling. Alt et al. (2022b) focused on several precursors of openness necessary to provide effective online counseling: preference for communicating emotions online, identification of the advantages of emotional expressiveness in providing online counseling, innovative behavior, creativity, and future problem-solving and thinking skills. The study focused on determining which constructs contribute to students' willingness to provide online counseling. The sample included 277 undergraduate students (future counselors and healthcare professionals) who filled out questionnaires. Data were analyzed using Partial Least Squares Structural Equation Modeling. The findings pointed to the centrality of students' preference for communicating their emotions online in explaining their openness to engaging in this form of counseling. Accordingly, the researchers suggested encouraging students to be open to providing counseling online. They also underscored the need to adjust the curriculum to better reflect the intensive changes within the fields of counseling and eHealth that necessitate shifting from face-to-face skills to online settings.

With respect to intrapersonal competencies, several studies have stressed the importance of cultivating skills such as self-regulation and reflection. Alt and

Naamati-Schneider (2021b) viewed self-regulation of learning as one of the key capabilities deemed essential for the healthcare system and its workers to cope successfully with current challenges. According to these researchers, healthcare curricula are increasingly called upon to support self-regulation as a central learning outcome. In view of the scarcity of relevant publications describing how students in medicine and other healthcare professions regulate their learning, they set out to design and assess problem-based learning using digital concept mapping in an online course and to evaluate the set of connections between this intervention and self-regulation of learning among health management students. One hundred students enrolled in a program for management of health service organizations were given a poorly structured problem relevant to their course content (accreditation within hospitals) and asked to argue for or against implementation of the accreditation process. The participants were asked to offer five arguments to establish their point by using *Mindomo*, a popular digital platform for designing concept maps. They were given predefined criteria that allowed them to self-assess their maps. Data for the analysis were collected by two measurements—concept mapping for the problem-based learning scale and the online self-regulated learning scale—and were then analyzed by Partial Least Squares Structural Equation Modeling. The findings showed that students' initial online self-regulation was lower than at the end of the intervention. Moreover, two self-regulation sub-factors—goal-setting and task strategies—were positively linked to students' perceptions of the intervention. After the intervention, the analyses showed an increase in four online self-regulation sub-factors: goal-setting, task strategies, environment structuring, and time management. The researchers concluded that teachers must recognize and account for different types of learners and encourage and scaffold students' effective use of self-regulation strategies. Learners with low levels of self-regulation may fail to see the advantages of concept mapping in problem-solving activities. When these teaching and learning tools are combined with advanced technology in an online course that encourages active learning, students in the medical and health management professions are able to develop and acquire self-directed learning abilities.

Alt et al. (2022c) focused attention on another intrapersonal competency, namely reflection. Reflective journal (RJ) writing has been recognized as an effective pedagogical tool for nurturing students' lifelong learning skills. Given the paucity of empirical work on the dimensionality of reflective writing, these researchers sought to qualitatively analyze students' RJ writing and design a generic reflection scheme for identifying dimensions of reflective thinking. Drawing on the theoretical scheme, they also sought to design and validate a questionnaire to measure students' perceptions of their reflective writing experiences. Their final aim was to quantitatively measure the link between perceived reflective writing and students' tendency to use RJs in their future careers and personal lives. This exploratory sequential research study comprised the following steps: First, the researchers collected experts' reviews and analyses of 1312 RJ entries. This step led to designing a theoretical scheme of reflective writing and a 31-item questionnaire used to gather data from 171 students (2nd year pre-service teachers and 3rd year health managers). Partial Least Squares analysis corroborated the structure of two timelines suggested by the theoretical scheme: reflections on the current course assignments and reflections related to the student's future development. Students' tendency to use reflective skills in their future professional lives was highly connected to their long-term reflections, including learning experiences linked to academic, professional, personal, and multicultural development. The validated generic scheme proposed in this study can be adapted and integrated into different curricula, where it may be used to infuse RJ instructional strategies into higher education curricula, improve the quality of reflection in student journals, and promote lifelong learning skills.

In examining interpersonal competencies such as collaboration, teamwork, and empathy/perspective taking, Alt and Naamati-Schneider (2021a) showed how collaboration in solving an authentic, value-laden problem can generate social perspective-taking among health management students. The activity described in their study, which included a moral dilemma, promoted socio-moral thinking skills and role-playing practices. The students examined a situation from another person's perspective and considered and evaluated the perspectives of others while engaging in social interactions and reading academic materials. This activity enabled them to understand the cognitive and emotional aspects of another individual. Incorporating an ethical dimension in the problem led to role-playing that may have contributed to the students' cognitive-moral development. Therefore, the authors suggested placing emphasis on equity in health education in an effort to strengthen the health system and its emergency responses during future public health crises.

According to Naamati-Schneider and Alt (2023a, 2023b), the use of tools such as Padlet appears to be effective in enhancing the collaboration skills of health management students. They designed an intervention program that employs online collaborative learning facilitated by Padlet to assess how flexible thinking while learning may affect how health management students evaluate their own learning performance. Two tools were used to collect data from 100 Israeli undergraduate students: *flexible thinking in learning* and *student perceptions of collaborative learning* via *Padlet.* The intervention program comprised several stages. First, the students discussed the pedagogic objective of using Padlet. Then they were given poorly structured problems related to the course content. Each group had to choose one problem and analyze it from three perspectives discussed in the course: healthcare provider, patient, and organization. Next, the students described their solutions by employing the shared knowledge base. They presented their final results in different formats using various technologies. The PLS-SEM analysis corroborated the hypothesis that students' flexible thinking makes a positive contribution to their perception of Padlet utilization. According to the empirical model, students who perceived themselves as more flexible were generally found to be more receptive to utilizing the proposed technological tool (Padlet) and hence tended to appreciate its use in facilitating collaborative learning platforms. This study underscores the important role played by flexible thinking in motivating managers and medical professionals to embrace innovative technologies or methods for teamwork. Such teamwork may enable them to weigh arguments, seek alternative solutions to authentic problems, and adjust their approaches effectively and collaboratively as new challenges emerge.

Soft skills were recently measured in the context of health management (Alt et al., 2023). These researchers underscored the importance of soft skills and their integration into educational system policy in higher education, particularly in view of the limited use of competency-based learning activities along with the widespread use of back-to-basics in many higher education systems. The study sought to examine how undergraduate students perceive the extent to which their faculty employed competency-based learning accompanied by formative assessment feedback techniques and to investigate how these methods affected their soft skill acquisition. Data were gathered from 303 Israeli undergraduate students, including health management students, and analyzed using Partial Least Squares—Structural Equation Modeling (PLS-SEM). The empirical model found that competency-based learning was positively connected to personal, social, and methodological soft skills. Moreover, formative assessment feedback demonstrated a high and positive association with competency-based learning, whereas the association between this factor and soft skills was low. These findings suggest that soft skills can be enhanced by constructivist learning activities that take place in meaningful and relevant vocational situations, accompanied by detailed feedback that is based on specific assessment criteria, provided in a timely manner, constructive, and aimed at reinforcing students' acquisition of soft skills.

Discussion

The importance of the 21CS outlined for healthcare managers cannot be overstated, as they play a crucial role in ensuring effective healthcare delivery and management. European countries' adoption of competency-based learning to bridge the gap between labor market demands and educational offerings highlights the critical need for such skills in healthcare management.

Firstly, cognitive competencies, such as understanding the healthcare environment and possessing business skills and knowledge, are fundamental. These competencies enable healthcare managers to navigate complex healthcare systems, understand funding mechanisms, and optimize organizational performance. Such knowledge is crucial for decision-making, strategic planning, and ensuring that healthcare services are both efficient and effective.

Secondly, intrapersonal competencies, including self-awareness, ethical conduct, and commitment to lifelong learning, are vital for personal and professional growth. Self-awareness allows managers to recognize their strengths and limitations, fostering a culture of continuous improvement and reflective leadership. Ethical conduct is essential in a field where decisions can have significant moral implications. Lifelong learning ensures that healthcare managers stay abreast of the latest developments in healthcare and management practices, thereby enhancing their effectiveness.

Thirdly, interpersonal competencies are critical in the healthcare environment. Skills like relationship management, communication, facilitation, and negotiation are indispensable for engaging with diverse stakeholders, including patients, families, and healthcare professionals. Effective communication and collaborative skills are essential for building trust, fostering teamwork, and ensuring that diverse perspectives are considered in decision-making processes.

Moreover, soft skills such as empathy, tolerance of stress, and interpersonal communication are integral to the healthcare setting. These skills contribute to better patient-therapist relationships, improved patient satisfaction and trust, and more accurate medical diagnoses and treatments. They also enhance team functioning, particularly under pressure, and promote a positive work environment, which is crucial in high-stress healthcare settings.

Integrating these competencies into health management studies through competency-based learning and assessment methods is crucial. It prepares healthcare managers to be more effective in their roles, ultimately leading to improved healthcare delivery and patient outcomes.

References

Alt, D., Boniel-Nissim, M., Naamati-Schneider, L., & Meirovich, A. (2022a). Precursors of openness to provide online counseling: The role of future thinking, creativity, and innovative behavior of future online therapists. *Frontiers in Psychology*. https://doi.org/10.3389/fpsyg.2022.848235

Alt, D., Naamati-Schneider, L., & Weishut, D. J. N. (2023). Competency-based learning and formative assessment feedback as precursors of college students' soft sills acquisition. *Assessment and Evaluation in Higher Education., 48*, 1901–1917. https://doi.org/10.1080/03075079.2023.2217203

Alt, D., & Naamati-Schneider, L. (2021a). Online argumentation-based learning aided by digital concept mapping during COVID-19: Implications for health management teaching and learning. *Health Education*. https://doi.org/10.1108/HE-12-2020-0125

Alt, D., & Naamati-Schneider, L. (2021b). Health management students' self-regulation and digital concept mapping in online learning environments. *BMC Medical Education*. https://doi.org/10.1186/s12909-021-02542-w

Alt, D., Naamati-Schneider, L., & Meirovich, A. (2022b). Future problem-solving practiced during Covid-19: Implications for health management students' e-Health literacy identity. *Frontiers in Psychology*. https://doi.org/10.3389/fpsyg.2022.829243

Alt, D., & Raichel, N. (2018). *Lifelong citizenship: Lifelong learning as a lever for moral and democratic values*. Brill and Sense Publishers.

Alt, D., & Raichel, N. (2020). Enhancing perceived digital literacy skills and creative self-concept through *gamified learning environments*: Insights from a longitudinal study. *International Journal of Educational Research*. https://doi.org/10.1016/j.ijer.2020.101561

Alt, D., & Raichel, N. (2021). *Equity and formative assessment in higher education: Advancing culturally responsive assessment*. Springer.

Alt, D., Raichel, N., & Naamati-Schneider, L. (2022c). Higher education students' reflective journal writing and lifelong learning skills: Insights from an exploratory sequential study. *Frontiers in Psychology*. https://doi.org/10.3389/fpsyg.2021.707168

American College of Healthcare Executives. (2022). *ACHE healthcare executive 2022 competencies assessment tool*. https://www.ache.org/-/media/ache/career-resource-center/cat-2022.pdf

Ammani, S., & Chitra, V. B. (2020). Blended learning of soft skills through life skills in an organization. *IUP Journal of Soft Skills, 14*(4), 7–11.

Back, A., Tulsky, J. A., & Arnold, R. M. (2020). Communication skills in the age of COVID-19. *Annals of Internal Medicine, 172*(11), 759–760. https://doi.org/10.7326/M20-1376

Barrera-Osorio, F., Kugler, A. D., & Silliman, M. I. (2020). *Hard and soft skills in vocational training: Experimental evidence from Colombia* (No. w27548). National Bureau of Economic Research.

Binkley, M., Erstad, O., Herman, J., Raizen, S., Ripley, M., Miller-Ricci, M., & Rumble, M. (2012). Defining twenty-first century skills. In P. Griffin & E. Care (Eds.), *Assessment and teaching of 21st century skills: Methods and approach* (pp. 17–66). Springer. https://doi.org/10.1007/978-94-007-2324-5_2

Bloom, B. S. (1956). *Taxonomy of educational objectives, handbook I: The cognitive domain.* David McKay.

Borge, M., & White, B. (2016). Toward the development of socio-metacognitive expertise: An approach to developing collaborative competence. *Cognition and Instruction, 34*(4), 323–360. https://doi.org/10.1080/07370008.2016.1215722

Bos–van den Hoek, D. W., Visser, L. N., Brown, R. F., Smets, E. M., & Henselmans, I. (2019). Communication skills training for healthcare professionals in oncology over the past decade: A systematic review of reviews. *Current Opinion in Supportive and Palliative Care, 13*(1), 33-45.

Carroll, J. B. (1993). *Human cognitive abilities.* Cambridge University Press.

Dimitrov, Y., & Vazova, T. (2020). Developing capabilities from the scope of emotional intelligence as part of the soft skills needed in the long-term care sector: presentation of pilot study and training methodology. *Journal of Primary Care & Community Health, 11.* https://doi.org/10.1177/2150132720906275

European Commission. (2018). *Commission staff working document accompanying the document proposal for a council recommendation on key competences for lifelong learning.* https://ec.europa.eu/

International Hospital Federation. (2015). *Leadership competencies for healthcare services managers.* https://www.ache.org/-/media/ache/about-ache/leadership_competencies_healthcare_services_managers.pdf

Karaca-Atik, A., Meeuwisse, M., Gorgievski, M., & Smeets, G. (2023). Uncovering important 21st-century skills for sustainable career development of social sciences graduates: a systematic review. *Educational Research Review, 39*, 100528.

Kahila, J., Valtonen, T., Tedre, M., Mäkitalo, K., & Saarikoski, O. (2020). Children's experiences on learning the 21st-century skills with digital games. *Games and Culture, 15*(6), 685–706. https://doi.org/10.1177/1555412019845592

Khaouja, I., Mezzour, G., Carley, K. M., & Kassou, I. (2019). Building a soft skill taxonomy from job openings. *Social Network Analysis and Mining, 9*(1), 1–19.

Lai, L., & Guo, F. (2018). Creating lifelong learners: Using project-based management to teach 21st Century skills. *Innovations in Education and Teaching International, 55*, 746–747.

Lepeley. M. T., Beutell, N. J., Abarca, N., & Majluf, N. (Eds.). (2021). *Soft skills for human centered management and global sustainability.* Routledge.

Markle, R., Brenneman, M., Jackson, T., Burrus, J., & Robbins, S. (2013). *Synthesizing frameworks of higher education student learning outcomes (ETS RR-13-22).* Educational Testing Service.

Naamati-Schneider, L., & Alt, D. (2023a). Online collaborative Padlet-mediated learning in health management studies. *Frontiers in Psychology, 14*, 1157621. https://doi.org/10.3389/fpsyg.2023.1157621

Naamati-Schneider, L., & Alt, D. (2023b). Enhancing collaborative learning in health management education: An investigation of Padlet-mediated interventions and the influence of flexible thinking. *BMC Medical Education, 23*(1), 846. https://doi.org/10.1186/s12909-023-04796-y

National Research Council. (2012). *Education for life and work: Developing transferable knowledge and skills in the 21st century.* National Academies Press.

Nehring, J. H., Charner-Laird, M., & Szczesiul, S. A. (2019). Redefining excellence: Teaching in transition, from test performance to 21st century skills. *NASSP Bulletin, 103*(1), 5–31. https://doi.org/10.1177/0192636519830772

Oliveri, M. E., & Mislevy, R. J. (2019). Introduction to "challenges and opportunities in the design of 'next-generation assessments of 21st century skills'" special issue. *International Journal of Testing, 19*, 97–102. https://doi.org/10.1080/15305058.2019.1608551

Organisation for Economic Co-operation and Development [OECD]. (2012). Better skills, better jobs, better lives: a strategic approach to skills policies. OECD.

Partnership for 21st Century Skills. (2014). *ICT literacy maps: Social studies map.* http://www.p21.org/images/stories/matrices/ICTmap_ss. pdf.

Redecker, C., Leis, M., Leendertse, M., Punie, Y., Gijsbers, G., & Kirschner, P. (2011). *The future of learning: Preparing for change: JRC-IPTS.* https://publications.jrc.ec.europa.eu

Rios, J. A., Ling, G., Pugh, R., Becker, D., & Bacall, A. (2020). Identifying critical 21st-century skills for workplace success: A content analysis of job advertisements. *Educational Researcher, 49*(2), 80–89. https://doi.org/10.3102/0013189X19890600

Sawyer, R. K. (2021). The dialogue of creativity: Teaching the creative process by animating student work as a collaborating creative agent. *Cognition and Instruction, 40*, 1–28. https://doi.org/10.1080/07370008.2021.1958219

Schunk, D. H., & Zimmerman, B. J. (Eds.). (1994). Self-regulation of learning and performance: Issues and educational applications. Lawrence Erlbaum Associates, Inc.

Schuster, C., Stebner, F., Leutner, D., & Wirth, J. (2020). Transfer of metacognitive skills in self-regulated learning: An experimental training study. *Metacognition and Learning, 15*(3), 455–477. https://doi.org/10.1007/s11409-020-09237-5

Shectman, N., DeBarger, A. H., Dornsife, C., Rosier, S., & Yarnall, L. (2013). Promoting grit, tenacity, and perseverance: Critical factors for success in the 21st century. Draft report for the US Department of Education. https://www.sri.com

Succi, C., & Canovi, M. (2020). Soft skills to enhance graduate employability: Comparing students and employers' perceptions. *Studies in Higher Education, 45*(9), 1834–1847. https://doi.org/10.1080/03075079.2019.1585420

Tindowen, D. J. C., Bassig, J. M., & Cagurangan, J. A. (2017). Twenty-first-century skills of alternative learning system learners. *Sage Open, 7*(3). https://doi.org/10.1177/2158244017726116

Tripathy, M. (2020). Relevance of soft skills in career success. *MIER Journal of Educational Studies Trends and Practices, 10*, 91–102.

Van Laar, E., van Deursen, A. J., van Dijk, J. A., & de Haan, J. (2020). Measuring the levels of 21st-century digital skills among professionals working within the creative industries: A performance-based approach. *Poetics, 81*, 101434. https://doi.org/10.1016/j.poetic.2020.101434

Vista, A. (2020). Data-driven identification of skills for the future: 21st-century skills for the 21st-century workforce. *SAGE Open, 10*(2), 2158244020915904.

Yao, M., Zhou, X. Y., Xu, Z. J., Lehman, R., Haroon, S., Jackson, D., & Cheng, K. K. (2021). The impact of training healthcare professionals' communication skills on the clinical care of diabetes and hypertension: A systematic review and meta-analysis. *BMC Family Practice, 22*(1), 1–23.

Zimmerman, B. J., & Moylan, A. R. (2009). Self-regulation: Where metacognition and motivation intersect. In D. J. Hacker, J. Dunlosky, & A. C. Graesser (Eds.), *Handbook of metacognition in education* (pp. 299–315). Routledge.

Zuma, S. K. (2021). Exploring the role of soft skills in advancing the employability of business graduates in Bangladesh. *Journal of International Business and Management, 4*(1), 10–18.

Part II
Cognitive Competencies

Chapter 4
Using Digital Concept Maps to Promote Argumentation Skills and Epistemological Beliefs Among Healthcare Management Students

Abstract Transforming traditional classroom activities into effective online learning experiences is a critical advancement in educational pedagogy. This chapter examines the application of constructivist pedagogy to problem-solving, specifically through the use of argumentation in distance learning contexts. It describes an undergraduate health system management course where a traditional face-to-face activity was replaced with an online argumentation-based learning exercise during the COVID-19 pandemic. The chapter explores the challenges and opportunities of this novel approach, incorporating digital concept mapping to enhance learning. The primary objective is to foster lifelong learning skills, such as higher-order thinking, critical thinking, and problem-solving abilities, among health management students.

Introduction

Cultivation of high-order thinking skills has been widely recognized as a crucial goal in health education (Medina et al., 2017). For this goal to be achieved, learning activities must be carefully designed both within individual courses and across curricula. According to Seymour-Walsh et al. (2020), the use of theoretically informed practices can help educators and course designers in the health professions explore innovative approaches for delivering high-quality education. Argumentation-based learning is considered to be one effective approach. Indeed, the prevalent assumption is that academia can play an important role in training doctors and healthcare professionals to develop and refine their argumentation skills.

The case study described in this chapter demonstrates how constructivist pedagogy can be applied to solve a problem through argumentation-based learning in a distance learning context. Specifically, the chapter examines the experiences of undergraduate health management students enrolled in an undergraduate Management of Health Service Organizations program during the COVID-19 pandemic, when an activity based on traditional face-to-face learning was replaced with an online argumentation-based learning activity that utilized digital concept mapping (CM). Using qualitative data analyses, the chapter examines the students' epistemological and ontological

L. Naamati-Schneider and D. Alt, *Technology and Competency-Oriented Learning*,
https://doi.org/10.1007/978-981-97-5771-8_4

standpoints to reveal their experiences with the activity. Furthermore, the chapter explores the key challenges posed by the online argumentation-based CM learning activity and the opportunities it offered for fostering lifelong learning skills, including high-order thinking, critical thinking, and problem-solving abilities.

Argumentation-Based Learning and High-Order Thinking Skills

The literature suggests various definitions of argumentation (Toulmin, 2003; Walton, 2006). Despite their differences, all these definitions see argumentation as a means for rationally resolving divergent opinions in critical discussions. Developing such decision-making skills is highly relevant in the context of global public health crises, when medical personnel must make rational and well-founded decisions in real time. According to Burkle's (2019) health crisis management model, these skills are essential requisites for meeting the strategic and operational requirements of mitigation, response, recovery, and rehabilitation during sudden-onset disasters and other time-limited crises.

In this chapter, the term "argument" refers to the artifacts created by students when asked to justify claims, whereas the term "argumentation" refers to the processes entailed in constructing these artifacts (Sampson & Clark, 2008). Based on the Piagetian equilibration model of socio-cognitive conflict (Piaget, 1985), such processes should provide learners the opportunity to review their ideas/beliefs, in turn motivating them to reconcile cognitive conflicts by explaining their views to the members of their group (Cheng, 2014).

One didactic method that bridges argumentation, domain-specific knowledge, and moral values is the Values and Knowledge Education (VaKE) approach (Weyringer et al., 2022). This approach exposes students to dilemmas relevant to their profession, clarifies the importance of their moral values and allows them to form independent opinions while encouraging dialogue and argumentation. This approach is largely informed by *social* cognition theory (Selman, 1980), which posits that a key factor in promoting social cognition is enhancing one's ability to understand the feelings and viewpoints of another person and to acknowledge that someone else's viewpoint may differ from one's own. Role-playing skills help people understand the cognitive and emotional attributes of others (i.e., moods, feelings, and attitudes).

According to Asterhan and Schwarz (2016), argumentation can improve high-order thinking skills that encompass conceptual, procedural, and metacognitive knowledge rather than being limited to factual knowledge. *Factual knowledge* pertains to the basic elements students must know to be sufficiently acquainted with a discipline or to solve problems (Anderson et al., 2001). Beyond the mere memorization of facts, *conceptual knowledge* refers to understanding similarities and patterns in factual knowledge and focuses on the interrelationships among the basic elements within a larger structure (Wilson, 2016). *Procedural knowledge* pertains to knowing "how" to do something, for example, how to use particular methods to achieve a specific learning goal (Anderson et al., 2001). *Metacognitive knowledge* encompasses knowledge of general strategies for learning and thinking and involves two main components: knowledge of cognition and regulation of cognition (Jacobs & Paris, 1987). Weinberger and Fischer (2006) maintain that these different types of knowledge can be achieved by encouraging students to construct arguments to justify their position.

The promotion of higher order thinking skills is considered an important learning outcome in health education. For example, Medina et al. (2017) maintain that metacognition is essential for confronting medical errors, which may occur, for example, because pharmacists do not always ask whether the doctor's orders make sense for the indications (i.e., metacognitive monitoring) or do not always check to make sure they entered information [in the computer database] correctly. Harris and Bacon (2019) underscored the advantages of active learning vs. passive learning in promoting cognitive skills among students in the healthcare profession. Based on their finding that student-centered learning techniques contribute more to lower- and higher-order cognition than passive learning methods, these researchers encourage educators to equalize instructional design to prioritize the needs of the student and the demand of the workforce.

Argumentation-Based Learning and Epistemological Beliefs

The epistemological beliefs of teachers and students regarding the nature of knowledge and learning may influence their approach to teaching and learning and the ways in which they make important instructional decisions and/or set their learning goals (Fives & Buehl, 2016). These beliefs are divided into teacher-centered instruction, in which the teacher is perceived as the sole transmitter of knowledge and the students as the knowledge recipients, and student-centered instruction, which gives priority to experience and active learning (Alt & Kapshuk, 2021). Students tend to rely on their previous experience and become accustomed to traditional learning methods, thus adopting an absolutist point of view (Kuhn et al., 2000) in which knowledge is composed of facts that are yet to be discovered.

Epistemological beliefs can be categorized into three distinct levels: absolutist, multiplist and evaluativist. On the *absolutist* level, knowledge is finite and unchanging and objective truth exists. On the *multiplist* level, knowledge is seen as inherently subjective and consisting not of facts but of opinions generated by humans that are indefinite and not subject to evaluation (Asterhan & Schwarz, 2016; Kuhn & Crowell, 2011). On highest level—the *evaluativist* level—individuals recognize the significance of weighing evidence and addressing contradictory claims (Kuhn et al., 2000).

Epistemological beliefs are often thought to be valuable precursors of student cognition, learning motivation, learning approaches, adaptive learning, and achievement (Greene et al., 2018). Nevertheless, despite broad acknowledgment that personal epistemology can influence students' beliefs about learning, research has not sufficiently addressed the use of educational programs in making an effective impact on individuals' epistemic beliefs.

Encouraging students to reach the *evaluativist* level, the highest level of epistemological beliefs, is considered a primary learning goal in health education (Cira et al., 2020; Hinneburg et al., 2020; Horntvedt et al., 2018). Evidence-based decision-making programs (Hinneburg et al., 2020) and evidence-based practices for physicians and for medical and nursing students (Cira et al., 2020) are considered imperative for ensuring patient safety. Students must be taught to recognize the value of weighing evidence through teaching and learning methods that encourage conscious use and application of a wide variety of knowledge sources. To do so requires formulating structured queries and searching trustworthy and reliable sources of evidence (Horntvedt et al., 2018). Yet although searching for evidence is considered a key competence for health practitioners, undergraduate programs continue to provide predominantly traditional, frontal classroom-teaching strategies whose abilities to foster the critical competencies required in real clinical contexts are limited (Park et al., 2020). Healthcare researchers recommend shifting education from merely providing decontextualized knowledge to a more innovative type of teaching that focuses on the use of scientific evidence to promote students' clinical reasoning and produce safe and effective healthcare outcomes.

The acquisition of higher epistemic beliefs appears to pose a challenge for clinicians; however, it may also provide opportunities for formulating important clinical questions, particularly during times of uncertainty (Naamati-Schneider & Alt, 2022). Cheng et al. (2020) reinforced this notion by focusing attention on the unique needs and concerns of healthcare students during the COVID-19 pandemic. These researchers highlighted the importance of designing learning activities to enhance students' critical thinking as a core skillset necessary for discovering facts and solving problems during times of crisis. Park et al. (2020) suggested web-based experiential learning strategies to improve engagement with and experience in learning environments aimed at helping students and clinicians recognize uncertainties in healthcare practices.

Web-Based Platforms for Argumentation-Based Learning

Research shows that several online settings support sharing, constructing, and representing arguments in multiple formats. For example, Alt and Naamati-Schneider (2021) noted a variety of recommended external knowledge representation tools designed to represent argumentation in Argumentation-Based Computer-Supported Collaborative Learning (ABCSCL) (e.g., Issue-Based Information Systems-IBIS). These tools can help learners clarify their arguments, argue more effectively, and find patterns of evidence.

According to Alt and Kapshuk (2021), even though computer-supported collaborative learning efforts appear to promote argumentation, further research is needed to establish this conjecture. To address this problem, the current study was the first to use a technology-enabled concept map method to facilitate argumentation processes. Concept maps (CM, Novak & Gowin, 1984) have been employed in education systems for over 30 years (Kinchin, 2014). Yet they have been used much less frequently to promote argumentation in higher education, and minimal attention has been paid to their use in online learning. Concept mapping is a learning method and educational tool that uses diagrammatic interrelationships between concepts that represent subject knowledge. CM should not merely list random textual information but rather should depict the structure of knowledge through propositional statements that illustrate the interrelationships between the given concepts in a map (Novak, 1981).

Through CM, students are expected to be able to transfer applied didactic objectives from the classroom to their clinical practice, where critical thinking and problem-solving skills are vital. This premise has been reinforced by several empirical studies demonstrating the benefits of CM used in concert with problem-based learning (PBL) for facilitating students' 21st-century skills. For example, Joshi and Vyas (2018) maintained that concept maps should be used in community medicine to solve epidemiological problems that focus on public health concepts, mathematical calculations, and "applied" interpretations. Similarly, Baig et al. (2016) examined the effectiveness of CM in medical students' academic problem-solving as well as in their declarative knowledge and their perceptions regarding CM. These researchers found that CM improved academic performance in problem-solving but not in declarative knowledge. Students' perceptions of the effectiveness of CM were positive. Another benefit of using CM is that it fosters students' ability to self-regulate their learning (Naderifar, 2018). Nevertheless, while concept maps have been shown to be an effective tool for facilitating students' critical thinking, research is still lacking on what CMs contribute to students' self-regulation abilities in face-to-face or online courses.

The literature surveyed above shows the potential of argumentation-based learning supported by digital CM to enhance students' lifelong learning skills (e.g., domain knowledge, critical thinking, problem-solving skills, and self-regulation abilities) and to shape their epistemic beliefs. In the current study we sought to discover how this innovative pedagogy can be employed online by analyzing the reflective journals of 65 students enrolled in a Management of Health Service Organizations program. To examine how the participants perceived the activity and its outcomes, we applied thematic analysis to the qualitative data by searching for themes and patterns pointing to different epistemological and ontological standpoints.

Designing Argumentation-Based Learning Supported by Digital CM

Values and Knowledge Education (VaKE, Weyringer et al., 2022) is a useful teaching tool that combines morality and values-centered education with knowledge content and stresses social behavior and the development of critical thinking in a PBL environment. In this study, the participants were third-year undergraduates pursuing degrees in healthcare systems management. We employed the VaKE approach to design a problem centered on accreditation issues, which was relevant to the course content. The 'Accreditation' process involves an external evaluation of healthcare organizations to assess their compliance with quality standards aimed at improving patient care. While its benefits are supported by limited research, accreditation drives positive changes in hospitals, leading to structural and cultural improvements, promoting standardized work processes, and enhancing organization and management practices. However, challenges like resource scarcity, limited manpower, and inadequate funding exist.

In this study, students were tasked with debating the implementation of an accreditation process in hospitals. The activity was structured into two phases. In the first phase, students individually or in groups used a concept map to outline five arguments supporting their stance. In the second phase, they applied course knowledge to gather evidence supporting their arguments and linked ethical values to at least two of these arguments. They then compared their arguments for similarities or differences using Mindomo, a concept mapping platform. Criteria for assessing the maps were provided in advance.

Students were asked to reflect on their learning process throughout the activity and record their thoughts in a reflective journal. They wrote about the development of their arguments from initial to more complex stages, the challenges faced, and the insights gained. Using reflective prompts (Alt et al., 2022), such as "Describe the main challenges" and "Describe what worked well," they were encouraged to engage in deep thinking about their experiences. Entries typically ranged from eight to ten paragraphs.

This study used thematic analysis to identify and report on additional themes emerging from the data. This approach is highly flexible and provides a rich and detailed account of data with only a few prescriptions and procedures. It is a practical, effective technique recommended for examining the viewpoints of different participants and summarizing key features of a large data set. Table 4.1 describes the stages in program implementation.

Table 4.1 Program stages

Stage	Students' role	Lecturer's role	Learning product
First stage	1. Group decision in favor of or against accreditation 2. Write down five arguments upon which you based your decision (without providing supportive evidence)	1. Presenting the dilemma 2. Presenting the task: Students must decide in favor of or against accreditation and write down five arguments upon which they based their decision 3. Technical guidance in using the Mindomo program/platform	Concept map showing the students' decision with five supporting arguments

(continued)

Table 4.1 (continued)

Stage	Students' role	Lecturer's role	Learning product
Second stage	1. Searching for information in support of the argument 2. Connecting at least two arguments to relevant ethical values 3. Describing the differences and similarities between the various arguments	1. 5–6 lessons about the dilemma, its implementation, and its repercussions 2. Guidance in constructing an argument and an opposing argument; importance of assessing information and ways of examining its reliability 3. Presenting the task: relating to the dilemma; basing arguments on reliable sources; locating ideological aspects and connections between arguments 4. Index for assessing quality of the concept map, including criteria for self-evaluation	Concept map representing the decision, the arguments, and at least two points of similarities or differences between arguments
After the first stage and throughout the second stage (optional)	Writing a reflective journal about personal learning processes and progress in designing the concept map, describing experiences, opportunities, and challenges accompanying the learning process	Students were not given any focused questions in this study, but only general ones, such as "Describe your experiences during the learning process". This enabled them to write freely about their learning processes	Students' reflective journals: average length 1000–1500 words in 7–8 paragraphs

Argumentation-Based Learning Supported by Digital CM: Students' Points of View

Analysis of the students' reflective journals yielded six categories: (1) from intuitive to evidence-based learning; (2) exposure to different perspectives; (3) domain-based knowledge (including factual, conceptual, procedural, and metacognitive knowledge); (4) from surface to deep learning; (5) prior knowledge and experience; and (6) values and knowledge.

From Intuitive to Evidence-Based Learning

During the learning process, the students underwent a perceptual epistemic change regarding learning and knowledge acquisition. At the beginning the students had no previous knowledge of the topic, so they used their intuition in building the first concept map. In seeking to provide a basis for their arguments, the students pursued many directions. Thus they were exposed to a complex reality about the topic that either contradicted or supported their initial point of view. Their journey toward understanding and acquiring firmly establishing knowledge began with their personal feelings and intuition in building the first map. In constructing the second map, they began to understand that they must establish the facts before making rational decisions. Shira, who participated in these activities, described her growing understanding as follows (Please note that pseudonyms are used throughout to maintain the privacy of the students):

> At the beginning of the assignment my understanding and arguments regarding accreditation were simple and not comprehensive or deep. After looking for material and reading information and articles, my opinions became stronger and my arguments and the basis for them became more complex and interesting. Accreditation poses obligations in all matters connected with people's health and bodies. Supervision of health has a major impact in the various organizations. Many articles cited testimonies and provided genuine evidence that strengthened my arguments and information. In addition, implementation of the accreditation code among patients and caregivers has led to improvements in the quality and level of patient treatment and service. Yet despite the code's many advantages, there are also many disadvantages and difficulties that challenge the healthcare system and exert a great deal of pressure on.

Other students noted that in preparing the second map, they were strongly committed to providing evidence-based arguments. They expressed a keen desire to find a concise and precise basis for their arguments that would confirm their confidence in their position. This was not easy for them, as it required extensive searching for and reading articles in Hebrew and English. The participants were determined not to compromise the quality of their sources to ensure that their arguments were supported by reliable literature that would not be easily contested. They diligently searched for articles that were not only closely aligned with their arguments but also provided additional advantages to accreditation. They went beyond the assignment's requirements and added supplementary secondary arguments to further strengthen their position.

In reviewing the literature, the participants also came across disadvantages that argued against accreditation. Yet they did not shy away from a balanced presentation of these disadvantages alongside the advantages. They attempted to compare the costs and the benefits by weighing the pros and cons of accreditation. Their commitment to finding precise and reliable evidence to support their arguments and their thorough exploration of both advantages and disadvantages showcased their dedication to thorough and comprehensive research.

Exposure to Different Perspectives

During the assignment, the students were given an opportunity to reexamine their ideas/beliefs. They sought to reconcile their cognitive conflict by explaining their views to the other members of their group. The discrepancy between what they know and what other people thinks often caused them to doubt the validity of their point of view, as expressed by Rina:

> All the members of the team participated in the discussion to clarify our argument by expressing their understanding from different viewpoints. This made me understand that there are different ways of looking at the same value. The discussion yielded a result that was acceptable to all team members. The map provided us a systematic view of all the ideas of the team members. The activity helped us because it enabled us to read opposing views about accreditation. We read articles in favor of accreditation, researched the topic thoroughly, and asked medical professionals about the issue. (My friend and I are interns in the delivery room at Hadassah Hospital Ein Karem and we learned from the staff there.) Working together with the group members also helped us formulate a concise opinion.

By adding secondary arguments and rationale to the first map, the participants became exposed to different ways of thinking and interpretations. The analysis showed that some of the participants' arguments were based on their own unique perspective and logic. Some of the secondary arguments they encountered did not seem to be directly connected to the issue at hand, and they struggled to understand the rationale behind these arguments. This observation reflected the diverse perspectives within the group, showing how the individuals member brought their own unique viewpoints and thought processes to the table.

The participants also highlighted the advantages of brainstorming with the other members of their group about the related implications and values. They welcomed the opportunity to "see different ways of thinking" and be exposed to how their colleagues related to the connections between the selected values. The differing points of views and values among the students necessitated finding points of agreement. As shown in the reflective journals, the group dynamics played a significant role in shaping the participants' arguments and perspectives. The diverse ways of thinking, interpretations, and values among the group members added depth and complexity to the mapping and highlighted the importance of collaborative discussions and finding common ground among differing viewpoints.

Some participants noted that the assignment encouraged them to take an interest in the opposing argument. They explained that the assignment had "compelled" them to investigate aspects that contradicted their initial assumption. Some entries in the reflective journals indicated that the participant's perspective towards accreditation had shifted during the assignment. For example, Iris mentioned that she was initially opposed to accreditation, but the majority opinion of her group members who favored accreditation convinced her to change her mind. She reflected on how her initial negative opinion may have been influenced by budgetary concerns or hearsay from nurses who viewed accreditation as a farce. Yet as she delved more deeply into the assignment and found articles in favor of accreditation, her perspective began to change. Gal had a similar experience:

> I developed many mixed feelings about accreditation. At first, I was opposed to implementing accreditation in hospitals, but now my feelings are divided. Considering the minor "research" we conducted on the topic, I also saw a lot of positive points about accreditation, such as improved service, relating to quality indexes, and relating to patients' viewpoints. These are important and result in fewer medical errors. This led me to reconsider my opinion, but not completely.

Some participants wrote that their perceptions was challenged during an ethics lesson when a guest lecturer revealed that there was no significant difference between accredited and non-accredited hospitals in the rate of medical errors or infections. This revelation made them question the validity and benefits of accreditation. They came to the conclusion that if accreditation is implemented honestly and with proper resources it has many advantages, but otherwise it may be unnecessary. The analysis reflects the participants' evolving perspective on accreditation, which was influenced by their group dynamics, research findings, and guest lectures. Their ability to reflect critically and reassess their initial opinion highlights the importance of evidence-based decision-making and the need to consider multiple perspectives in complex issues such as accreditation.

Domain-Based Knowledge

The literature review suggests that in addition to improving factual knowledge, argumentation can improve conceptual, procedural, and metacognitive knowledge. Analysis of the students' journals revealed that beyond merely supporting factual knowledge, in many cases the assignment helped students begin thinking on a higher level, along a continuum from conceptual to procedural to metacognitive knowledge.

Factual knowledge

The students reported that doing the assignment exposed them to vast amounts of knowledge. The assignment enriched their world of knowledge and expanding their understanding about the advantages and disadvantages of accreditation. As described by Gil, this stage helped them begin to formulate the second map and marked the beginning of the road to establishing an argument:

> Doing an assignment on a topic such as accreditation, which can be explained in positive or negative terms, enriched my knowledge about the accreditation process being implemented in hospitals and helped me understand the factors influencing the quality of service hospitals provide. The research reflected the patients' point of view by examining everything patients undergo from the moment they enter the hospital until they are discharged or continue receiving treatment in the community. The hospital management receives feedback from patients. I am pleased that there is a process designed to improve the quality of treatment and service.

Conceptual knowledge

Conceptual knowledge was a recurrent theme in the students' reflective reports. This type of knowledge refers to patterns and interrelationships among the basic elements within a larger structure that enable them to function together, e.g., knowledge about similarities and patterns in factual knowledge elements. The students mainly emphasized what the CM contributed to their ability to organize their knowledge and identify the connections between arguments. Some recognized the advantages of using a map to arrange information, claiming that the visual organization of information on a map helped underscore the connections between different components, while also requiring them to focus on the main points of the arguments and present the material concisely and effectively. The participants highlighted the benefits of using a visual tool such as a map to convey complex information. The use of a map allowed for clear and structured representation of the connections and relationships between different components of the arguments, thus facilitating understanding and communication. This perspective indicates that the participants saw the visual format of a map as more effective and conducive to their learning and presentation style than a standard Word file, as described by Gabi:

> I can see the advantages of arranging information on a map. The map helps present information visually, emphasizes the connections between the various components, and obligates you to focus on the main points of the arguments and to present the material in a concise and effective way. I think that submitting a standard WORD file with the same arguments would have been less effective.

Sigal, a student with a severe attention deficit disorder, also praised the advantages of using a map for information organization and presentation. Her preference for a visual format such as a map emphasizes the importance of using different means of presenting information to enhance understanding and effectiveness in academic assignments or other contexts.

> I have a severe attention deficit disorder, and assembling the material in this way helped me a lot. I was unable to gain any logical understanding of the material until we arranged it on the map. It was difficult for me to understand how to assemble the map because I can comprehend the visual portion better. After we assembled the map, all the separate pieces of the puzzle came together. The arguments and their associated values were the parts that required the most thought and time. It took me a long time to understand how to do this from a technical standpoint. Only then was I able to delve more deeply into the data, thoroughly analyze the arguments, and find the connections between them. As I drew more connections and parts on the map, I was able to think about the topic more deeply.

Procedural knowledge

Procedural knowledge pertains to knowing "how" to do something, for example, how to use particular methods to achieve a specific learning goal. Some of the participants indicated that the activity had taught them to use a new tool, which they could apply in the future to solve similar problems in their professional work. The tool enabled them to formulate objectives while also developing critical thinking. Lina expressed this as follows:

> The way the message was presented was interesting and challenging. We were exposed to new possibilities for conveying our message while pursuing our academic degree. I am certain these new programs will benefit me in the future in staff meetings at work. I can use them to define organizational objectives, prepare annual summaries, or present projects in a way that observers can understand.

The participants also highlighted how the use of the map as a learning tool offered them a new way to learn. It was their first time working with the application, and they found it helpful in expanding their thinking. They mentioned that they could use the application in the future to formulate ideas more clearly and comprehensively when presenting a topic or dilemma. The participants expressed their intention to utilize the map tool to present all arguments in favor or against a particular topic or to support their viewpoints. They indicated that accreditation is of utmost importance and they are committed to follow up on it more carefully in the future to ensure that their patients receive proper treatment.

These comments reflect the participants' recognition of the benefits of the accreditation process in healthcare, as well as their positive experience using the map as a learning tool. Their eagerness to apply the skills and knowledge gained from this activity in their future endeavors demonstrates their enthusiasm for ongoing learning and improvement in their professional practice. The following statement by Gali demonstrates the students' positive attitude towards the activity and their intention to utilize the skills they learned in their future work:

> For me, the map offered a new way to learn. This was the first time I worked with this application. It helped me by providing tools to expand my thinking. If I want to present a topic or a dilemma in the future, I'll be able to use the program we learned to convey my ideas more clearly and comprehensively. I can use it to present all the arguments in favor of or against my point of view.

Other participants noted that they learned the importance of searching for information to achieve a specific learning goal. The activity forced them to embark on a comprehensive search for information, including information that contradicted their arguments. This provided them a clearer picture of the issue and enabled them to better substantiate their positions regarding accreditation, as noted by Riki:

> The assignment helped us understand what accreditation is. During our first lesson with you, we didn't understand the meaning of accreditation and we couldn't even pronounce the word correctly, but there is no doubt that today we know a lot more. Searching for more articles about this topic forced us to read more and more about different opinions, both pro and con. Apparently, this topic has stimulated a lot of dialogue and provoked numerous opinions.

Metacognitive knowledge

The students described how the activity helped them self-regulate their learning, in line with the principles of the theory of self-regulation for learning. David's reflections echo the key tenets of this theory as he navigated through the challenges of the activity:

> I felt I was acquiring a new skill, over and above receiving a grade in the course. The search for information about the topic in general and the use of the concept map in particular offered me a challenge. At times I felt this was difficult for me and that things were not clear, that I didn't understand, and that I didn't have enough time.

David's awareness of his own cognitive and emotional states as well as his metacognitive monitoring of his learning process exemplified the self-regulatory processes outlined by the theory. He further acknowledged the importance of external support in his self-regulation, stating, "However, with the help of my teammates and the lecturer who devoted her time to explain things, I was able to attain the course objective." This statement highlights the role of social and environmental factors in self-regulated learning. David also expressed a sense of achievement and mastery, which are central to the theory of self-regulation for learning: "I think I became more proficient with the material we had to find and examine. I also acquired a new tool I can use to present material about various topics and formulate an opinion." David's reflections demonstrate his application of self-regulatory strategies, his metacognitive awareness, and the impact of external support on his learning process, in line with the core principles of the theory of self-regulation for learning.

One of the most valuable tools in promoting self-regulation for learning was the table of criteria used to evaluate the concept map that the students constructed together with the instructors. Ifat stated:

> The criteria for evaluating the map were clear and easy to understood and helped me see how my map was supposed to be constructed and what it should look like. The criteria helped me ensure that the map's contents would be of the highest possible quality and would be interconnected either directly or indirectly. The criteria helped me understand what was expected of me. They gave me the confidence to understand that even though the task was relatively complex and even though I had never used the program before, I was headed in the right direction, I knew what to improve and how to progress.

From Surface to Deep Learning

To complete the assignment and resolve the dilemma, the students had to use various research strategies. Unlike in the pursuit of factual knowledge, which is based on primary research, the students were required to research an existing reality to form an opinion about the topic. Their research journey provided them a better understanding of the issues and encouraged them to examine the topic more deeply. Sarit noted:

> My position remained in favor of accreditation. Indeed, it became stronger as we *deepened* the search for material on the internet. We saw the significance of the hospital's growing reputation and its international standing. We also learned about how the hospital motivated its employees as well as about cultural and linguistic accessibility in healthcare organizations and about the Hippocratic Oath. The existence of the accreditation process which seeks to raise the level of Israeli hospitals to an international standard, reflects the hospitals' objective of saving human lives. This objective can be accomplished through all the options mentioned above.

As Ruth aptly stated, "The activity definitely helped us gain a deeper understanding of the topic of accreditation in hospitals." This statement is in line with the principles of deep learning theory, according to which processing and active engagement with the material leads to better retention and comprehension. Actively processing and internalizing material, whether by mapping concepts or using other presentation methods, facilitates better understanding and longer retention. Ruth's observation that "anyone who processes material will remember it and understand it better" underscores the significance of active engagement in learning. By actively processing and integrating material, we can enhance our understanding and retain knowledge for an extended period of time, as Ruth astutely pointed out.

Prior Knowledge and Experience

The theme of prior knowledge and experience refers to students' ability to incorporate their own background knowledge. The participants reported that the opportunity they were given to apply prior knowledge helped them learn. Some drew upon prior knowledge acquired throughout their lifetime, which they found beneficial when proposing a solution to the problem. For example, Shira had previous experience working in a hospital. This experience served as an additional information source for understanding the issue of accreditation. Despite this, she still needed more supportive evidence to consolidate her opinion into a well-established argument:

> I did my national service in the outpatient clinic of the Hematology Department at Shaare Zedek Hospital in Jerusalem in 2017. At the time the hospital was preparing for accreditation examinations. The women doing national service were mobilized together with the doctors, nurses, and management to ensure that the hospital met the requirements. Even before we began working on the map, I felt I was already familiar with the issue and was opposed to the accreditation examination in its present form. My opinion was based both on what we learned in class and on my previous personal experience. As we progressed from the first map to the second and read more articles, I began to understand that my viewpoint was narrow. I have now acquired more information that has provided me a more comprehensive view of accreditation.

Values and Knowledge

One of the tasks in the assignment was to find values connected to the arguments or to the supporting evidence. This process is based on an approach known as values and knowledge education (VaKE), according to which a specific field of knowledge can be taught by underscoring the relationships between theory and its practical application, including dialogue regarding a relevant moral dilemma. Confronting a dilemma entails teamwork and discussing the pros and cons of problem-solving alternatives, while considering values and finding information necessary to establish arguments. For some of the participants, this assignment focused on connecting the learning material to their world of values, as explained for example by Shirly:

> One of the most important sentences on the map was "Whoever saves one life saves an entire world." This sentence has great significance for me and for the hospitals. It is a sufficient reason for them to meet the required parameters for accreditation. From their standpoint, if they saved one person, they save an entire world.

Yet many students had trouble seeing how their set of arguments and the materials they found were compatible with values. They initially expressed these difficulties in terms of an inability to define the values, to assess which values were connected to the material, and ultimately to determine the connection between values and the arguments. According to Yoram:

> The stage about values was difficult for all the members of the group, and particularly for me. It took us (a long) time to determine exactly how values should be defined. We finally proposed values that we felt were important. The accreditation process helps in implementing these values optimally and effectively. We proposed some values that accreditation promotes and others that it is liable to harm.

Discussion

This chapter has attempted to show how health management students can engage in constructivist learning online. It demonstrates how the promotion of argumentation-based learning with digital CM can elicit new and different beliefs and conceptions of learning and knowledge, guide students from intuitive to evidence-based learning, expose them to different perspectives while encouraging deep learning based on their prior knowledge and experience, and nurture a value-laden educational approach.

At the outset, the students based their arguments primarily on intuition and "all or nothing" definitions offered during short lectures at the beginning of the course, thus exhibiting their belief in the existence of absolute truths. As the learning progressed, the students were exposed to an array of different viewpoints. They began to recognize the complexity of the topic, thus achieving a higher level of epistemological belief where knowledge is seen as inherently subjective and generated by human minds. Finally, the requirement that they base their arguments on facts brought them to the higher epistemological level of *evaluativism*, where they recognized the significance of weighing evidence and addressing contradictory knowledge claims (Kuhn et al., 2000). Students who undergo an epistemic change during constructivist practices will demonstrate an ability to alter preconceived epistemic beliefs regarding how the health professions should be taught and how critical thinking skills should be attained.

The activity also promoted socio-moral thinking skills and role-playing practices. The students examined the situation from the perspectives of others and considered and evaluated these perspectives while engaging in social interactions and reading academic materials (Kim et al., 2018). This practice is related to social cognition theory (Selman, 1980) and role-playing skills that enable a person to understand the cognitive and emotional aspects of another. In line with the VaKE approach, incorporating an ethical dimension into the problem led to role-playing, which may have contributed to the students' cognitive-moral development. Learning initiatives that nurture socio-moral thinking have the potential to produce a generation of professional practitioners who aspire to prioritize solutions dedicated to collaboration and social justice (Siry, 2020).

In the field of health management education, transitioning from conventional teaching methods to more progressive, evidence-based instructional techniques appears essential for cultivating the vital competencies needed in actual clinical environments. Emphasizing evidence-based decision-making equips students with the skills to critically engage with a variety of knowledge sources, fostering a deeper understanding of patient safety and clinical decision-making. This educational approach encourages students to formulate structured queries and apply reliable information in practical settings, which is essential for navigating the complexities of modern healthcare.

The transition to experiential and technology-based learning strategies may enhance student engagement and provides a hands-on approach to learning. These methods are particularly effective in fostering critical thinking and clinical reasoning skills, enabling students to recognize and address uncertainties in healthcare practices. The adaptability and problem-solving skills honed through these methods are particularly crucial in times of crisis, such as during the COVID-19 pandemic.

Innovative teaching methods that focus on the application of scientific evidence and experiential learning are key to producing competent health management professionals. Such educational approaches equip students with the necessary tools to think critically, make informed decisions, and contribute to safe and effective healthcare outcomes. As healthcare environments become increasingly complex, the ability to adapt, learn continuously, and apply evidence-based knowledge becomes indispensable for future healthcare leaders. This evolution in teaching strategies ensures that health management students are not only well-versed in theoretical knowledge but are also prepared to apply this knowledge effectively in real-world scenarios.

References

Alt, D., & Kapshuk, Y. (2021). Argumentation-based learning with digital concept mapping and college students' epistemic beliefs. *Learning Environments Research, 25*(3), 687–706. https://doi.org/10.1007/s10984-021-09385-8

Alt, D., & Naamati-Schneider, L. (2021). Online argumentation-based learning aided by digital concept mapping during COVID-19: Implications for health management teaching and learning. *Health Education, 122*, 18–36. https://doi.org/10.1108/HE-12-2020-0125

Alt, D., & Raichel, N. (2018). *Lifelong citizenship: Lifelong learning as a lever for moral and democratic values*. Brill and Sense Publishers.

Alt, D., Raichel, N., & Naamati-Schneider, L. (2022). Higher education students' reflective journal writing and lifelong learning skills: Insights from an exploratory sequential study. *Frontiers in Psychology*. https://doi.org/10.3389/fpsyg.2021.707168

Anderson, L. W., Krathwohl, D. R., Airasian, P. W., Cruiskshank, K. A., Mayer, R. E., Pintrich, P. R., Raths, J., & Wittrock, M. C. (2001). *A taxonomy for learning, teaching, and assessing*. Longman.

Asterhan, C. S., & Schwarz, B. B. (2016). Argumentation for learning: Well-trodden paths and unexplored territories. *Educational Psychologist, 51*(2), 164–187.

Baig, M., Tariq, S., Rehman, R., Ali, S., & Gazzaz, Z. J. (2016). Concept mapping improves academic performance in problem solving questions in biochemistry subject. *Pakistan Journal of Medical Sciences Quarterly, 32*(4), 801–805.

Burkle, F. M., Jr. (2019). Challenges of global public health emergencies: Development of a health-crisis management framework. *The Tohoku Journal of Experimental Medicine, 249*(1), 33–41. https://doi.org/10.1620/tjem.249.33

Cheng, S. C. (2014). *Effects of socio-cognitive conflicts on group cognition and group performance* (Unpublished doctoral dissertation). Harvard Graduate School of Education.

Cheng, Y. C., Huang, L. C., Yang, C. H., & Chang, H. C. (2020). Experiential learning program to strengthen self-reflection and critical thinking in freshmen nursing students during COVID-19: A quasi-experimental study. *International Journal of Environmental Research and Public Health, 17*(15), 5442.

Cira, M. K., Tesfay, R., Zujewski, J. A., Sinulingga, D. T., Aung, S., Mwakatobe, K., Lasebikan, N., Nkegoum, B., Duncan, K., & Dvaladze, A. (2020). Promoting evidence-based practices for breast cancer care through web-based collaborative learning. *Journal of Cancer Policy, 25*, 100242. https://doi.org/10.1016/j.jcpo.2020.100242

Fives, H., & Buehl, M. M. (2016). Teachers' beliefs, in the context of policy reform. *Behavioral and Brain Sciences, 3*, 114–121. https://doi.org/10.1177/2372732215623554

Greene, J. A., Cartiff, B. M., & Duke, R. F. (2018). A meta-analytic review of the relationship between epistemic cognition and academic achievement. *Journal of Educational Psychology, 110*(8), 1084. https://psycnet.apa.org/doi/10.1037/edu0000263

Harris, N., & Bacon, C. E. W. (2019). Developing cognitive skills through active learning: A systematic review of health care professions. *Athletic Training Education Journal, 14*(2), 135–148. https://doi.org/10.4085/1402135

Horntvedt, M. E. T., Nordsteien, A., Fermann, T., & Severinsson, E. (2018). Strategies for teaching evidence-based practice in nursing education: A thematic literature review. *BMC Medical Education, 18*(1), 172. https://doi.org/10.1186/s12909-018-1278-z

Hinneburg, J., Hecht, L., Berger-Höger, B., Buhse, S., Lühnen, J., & Steckelberg, A. (2020). Development and piloting of a blended learning training programme for physicians and medical students to enhance their competences in evidence-based decision-making. *Zeitschrift Für Evidenz, Fortbildung und Qualität Im Gesundheitswesen, 150*, 104–111. https://doi.org/10.1016/j.zefq.2020.02.004

Jacobs, J. E., & Paris, S. G. (1987). Children's metacognition about reading: Issues in definition, measurement, and instruction. *Journal of Educational Psychology, 22*, 255–278.

Joshi, U., & Vyas, S. (2018). Assessment of perception and effectiveness of concept mapping in learning epidemiology. *Indian Journal of Community Medicine, 43*(1). http://ezproxy.kinneret.ac.il:2057/10.4103/ijcm.IJCM_375_16

Kim, H. Y., LaRusso, M. D., Hsin, L. B., Harbaugh, A. G., Selman, R. L., & Snow, C. E. (2018). Social perspective-taking performance: Construct, measurement, and relations with academic performance and engagement. *Journal of Applied Developmental Psychology, 57*, 24–41. https://psycnet.apa.org/doi/10.1016/j.appdev.2018.05.005

Kinchin, I. M. (2014). Concept mapping as a learning tool in higher education: a critical analysis of recent reviews. *The Journal of Continuing Higher Education, 62*, 39–49. https://psycnet.apa.org/doi/10.1016/j.appdev.2018.05.005

Kuhn, D., Cheney, R., & Weinstock, M. (2000). The development of epistemological understanding. *Cognitive Development, 15*(3), 309–328.

Kuhn, D., & Crowell, A. (2011). Dialogic argumentation as a vehicle for developing young adolescents' thinking. *Psychological Science, 22*, 545–552. https://doi.org/10.1177/0956797611402512

Medina, M. S., Castleberry, A. N., & Persky, A. M. (2017). Strategies for improving learner metacognition in health professional education. *American Journal of Pharmaceutical Education, 81*(4). https://doi.org/10.5688%2Fajpe81478

Naamati-Schneider, L., & Alt, D. (2022). Implications of dilemma-based learning and the use of argumentation aided by digital concept mapping during COVID-19 for Health Management students' epistemological and ontological perceptions and thinking levels. *Zman Hinuch (time for Education), 7*, 21–42. (Hebrew).

Naderifar, A. (2018). The comparative effect of concept mapping and vocabulary notebook keeping on Iranian EFL learners' self-regulation in vocabulary learning. *Cogent Education, 5*(1). https://doi.org/10.1080/2331186X.2018.1491782

Novak, J. (1981). Applying learning psychology and philosophy to biology teaching. *The American Biology Teacher, 43*(1), 12–20.

Novak, J. D., & Gowin, D. B. (1984). *Learning how to learn.* Cambridge University Press.

Park, M., Jeong, M., Lee, M., & Cullen, L. (2020). Web-based experiential learning strategies to enhance the evidence-based-practice competence of undergraduate nursing students. *Nurse Education Today*, 104466. https://doi.org/10.1016/j.nedt.2020.104466

Piaget, J. (1975/1985). *The equilibration of cognitive structures: The central problem of intellectual development*. University of Chicago Press.

Sampson, V., & Clark, D. B. (2008). Assessment of the ways students generate arguments in science education: Current perspectives and recommendations for future directions. *Science Education, 92*, 447–472. https://doi.org/10.1002/sce.20276

Selman, R. L. (1980). *The growth of interpersonal understanding: Developmental and clinical analyses.* Academic Press.

Seymour-Walsh, A. E., Weber, A., & Bell, A. (2020). Pedagogical foundations to online lectures in health professions education. *Rural and Remote Health, 20*(2). https://doi.org/10.22605/rrh 6038

Siry, C. (2020). Science education during times of crisis: calling for reflections, responses, and forward thinking from the CSSE community. *Cultural Studies of Science Education, 15*(2), 317–322. https://doi.org/10.1007%2Fs11422-020-09985-5

Toulmin, S. E. (2003). *The uses of argument.* Updated ed. Cambridge University Press (1st ed. 1958).

Walton, D. N. (2006). Examination dialogue: An argumentation framework for critically questioning an expert opinion. *Journal of Pragmatics, 38*(5), 745–777.

Weinberger, A., & Fischer, F. (2006). A framework to analyze argumentative knowledge construction in computer-supported collaborative learning. *Computers & Education, 46*(1), 71–95. https://doi.org/10.1016/j.compedu.2005.04.003

Weyringer, S., Patry, J. L., Pnevmatikos, D., & Børhaug, F. B. (2022). *The VaKE handbook: Theory and practice of values and knowledge education* (Vol. 18). Brill.

Wilson, L. O. (2016). Anderson and Krathwohl–Bloom's taxonomy revised. *Understanding the New Version of Bloom's Taxonomy.* Retrieved from https://quincycollege.edu/content/uploads/Anderson-and-Krathwohl_Revised-Blooms-Taxonomy.pdf

Chapter 5
Cultivating Future Thinking, Creativity, and Innovation Through E-Poster Engagement: Essential Competencies for Contemporary Healthcare Managers

Abstract In an era where creativity and innovative problem-solving are paramount, fostering these skills in health management education is crucial. This chapter explores the role of future problem-solving programs in enhancing flexible thinking and innovative problem-solving methods. It demonstrates the use of the Future Problem Solving (FPS) program in health management courses, where students engaged in a six-step process to tackle future challenges and propose practical solutions. The FPS program encouraged students to generate diverse solutions for complex problems, identify unknown factors, and establish connections among seemingly unrelated ideas. The chapter details the FPS technique and discusses its contribution to health management students' awareness of creative and innovative ideas applicable in health professions.

Introduction

As early as 1978 Torrance and Torrance pointed to an alarming trend: students are not sufficiently proactive in forecasting potential problems they may encounter in the future and in devising creative solutions to those problems. In an effort to curb this trend, they initiated the Future Problem Solving (FPS) program. Contemporary researchers (Azevedo et al., 2016; Treffinger et al., 2012) voiced similar concerns, contending that the fact that we live in uncertain times makes the need to delve into the future more important than ever. Consequently, students must be able to think critically, use thinking skills and innovative strategies in a variety of ways and adapt them to the changing reality.

Previous studies have shown the centrality of FPS programs in promoting learner creativity (Alzahrani et al., 2020; Dochy & Segers, 2018) in that such programs encourage skills relevant to flexible thinking and creative, fluent and innovative problem-solving (Alt & Raichel, 2018). Nevertheless, very little research has examined learning programs in higher education based on solving future problems. This chapter describes how the implementation of such a learning program in healthcare

L. Naamati-Schneider and D. Alt, *Technology and Competency-Oriented Learning*,
https://doi.org/10.1007/978-981-97-5771-8_5

management education helped learners think creatively and innovatively by making them more aware of future health problems.

Future Problem Solving Program

Torrance and Torrance (1978) initiated the FPS program in 1974 in the US. They contended that using analytical methods to solve problems is no longer practical because problems are becoming increasingly unpredictable. Hence, people must learn how to adapt to changes by means of creativity (Torrance & Cramond, 2002). Indeed, applying established rules and logical reasoning within the context of known information when solving a problem narrows down the potential solutions and excludes the innovative approaches needed to solve problems from a futuristic perspective. The FPS program was based on creative problem-solving and futurist thinking. Its overarching aims were to encourage young students to solve problems critically in hypothetical future situations, spark their creativity and improve their thinking skills (Azevedo et al., 2019).

The ability to solve future problems has become central in educational programs worldwide (Treffinger et al., 2012). These programs use authentic social problems that reflect concerns about contemporary trends that are likely to affect society in the future, and the solutions should provide ways for society to adapt to future situations. In such inquiry activities, students are encouraged to offer creative and innovative solutions to address the challenges at issue (Main et al., 2019). The problem can be related to any topic, for example, social and political issues or a business and technology theme based on future situations that is already relevant today.

FPS is based on futuristic thinking and the creative problem-solving method. It begins by identifying and defining a problem and ends by suggesting an effective and original solution (Azevedo et al., 2016). FPS incorporates six steps (Cramond, 2009; Torrance & Cramond, 2002): (1) identifying challenges in a future situation that is problematic or fuzzy; (2) selecting an underlying problem to be tackled; (3) generating possible solutions to the underlying problem without judgment; (4) generating and selecting evaluation criteria for the suggested solutions; (5) evaluating and ranking the possible solutions according to the criteria and choosing the best one; (6) developing an action plan to demonstrate how the solution will work to solve the underlying problem.

Thus far, FPS programs have primarily targeted children and adolescents, usually talented students from different age groups (Treffinger et al., 2021). The program's stated mission specifically targets young people and seeks to develop their ability to promote positive futures by creatively solving problems (Azevedo et al., 2016). FPS is considered a prominent educational process that spurs gifted students' imagination and encourages them to explore challenges and find solutions within a limited period of time (Kashani-Vahid et al., 2017). Because of the targeted age group, very little research has examined the program's application and effectiveness in higher education. For example, Vijayaratnam (2012) used a futuristic real-world scenario to engage budding engineers in a problem-solving task. The study measured the task's effectiveness in developing students' higher-order thinking, problem-solving and collaborative skills. The findings showed that using real-world tasks in small groups has the potential to help students relate theory to practice and to encourage them to build on sharable knowledge and apply it in real-world scenarios, thereby harnessing their higher-order thinking and team skills.

Problem Solving and Creativity

Creativity is often defined as the ability to produce ideas and products that are innovative, (i.e., original or unexpected) and useful (i.e., appropriate or meet task constraints, Runco & Jaeger, 2012). Mumford et al., (2009, p. 67) succinctly defined creativity as "the nature of thought processes and intellectual activity used to generate new insights or solutions to problems." Several studies have demonstrated the effectiveness of future thinking in developing creativity (Treffinger et al., 2021). For example, Treffinger et al. (2012) investigated the effectiveness of a program for solving future problems among high school students and showed how the program helped participants develop more vital images of their future, thus boosting their creative abilities. Similarly, Azevedo et al. (2019) explored an international program for solving future problems aimed at promoting creative, critical and future thinking among adolescents. The results showed that the program was more effective in enhancing students' creative skills compared to a control group. Learners who believe in their creativity tend to invest more in creative tasks and therefore solve problems that require creative thinking more effectively (Pretz & Nelson, 2017). This belief in creativity has been found to be related to creative behavior (Czerwonka & Karwowski, 2018) and creative achievements (Karwowski & Barbot, 2016).

In the context of healthcare, a great deal of research, although not centered specifically on FPS, has assessed the effectiveness of instructional interventions aimed at developing creativity, particularly in the context of creative problem-solving. Luu et al. (2019) claimed that within the healthcare sector, empirical research has largely defined creativity as an outcome that focuses on generating novel and useful ideas pertaining to products, services and processes. In this context, creativity is not simply about novelty but also involves identifying usefulness in ideas and solutions. Consequently, research has explored creative solutions to problems, creative strategies and creative modifications to job processes in both private and public sector organizations. In particular, creativity management has been suggested as an effective approach to broaden innovation practices within public organizations.

Creative outcomes can vary from minor adjustments in workflow, products or services (incremental creativity) to major breakthroughs and the development of new products, services or processes (radical creativity). Research suggests that creativity in the private sector tends to be more radical and strategic, whereas in the public sector creativity is often more incremental in nature (Lauring & Selmer, 2013). Clinicians, including physicians and nurses, can generate creative outcomes ranging from minor modifications to treatment or nursing protocols to the development of new treatment methods, techniques or nursing processes. Such novel and useful outcomes contribute to the effectiveness of treatment and nursing.

Team creativity refers to the joint generation of novel and useful ideas by a group of individuals, such as a department of clinicians in a hospital. Creativity enables teams to address problems and to seize opportunities by integrating diverse perspectives and viewpoints. In many organizations, particularly healthcare organizations, creative capital is considered to be the most valuable asset. The ability to leverage the creative potential of teams is crucial to the success of organizations and to their ability to adapt in the face of changing environmental forces (Luu et al., 2019).

Problem Solving and Innovation

Innovation is associated with the generation, promotion and implementation of ideas, and includes opportunities for adaptation (Zhou & Verburg, 2020). An innovation process often starts with a discovery or is triggered by a problem requiring an urgent response. This process leads to idea exploration and finding ways to improve products, services or processes. Ideas are then generated that offer solutions to the problems. This process includes gathering support by exhibiting enthusiasm and confidence about the innovation, followed by implementing, testing and modifying the idea.

Carr et al. (2016) specified two types of innovations. The first type involves goal-directed and problem-induced behavior that is prompted by the need to find a solution to a problem ("active" innovations). This type of innovation requires individuals to have experience and exhibit cognitive maturity. The second type of innovation, in contrast, is considered more incidental or accidental as it arises "not due to the need for a solution to a problem but as a result of situations offering chance, and scope for, novel behaviors" (p. 1513). Nevertheless, the authors claimed that this type of innovation cannot be learned and therefore cannot be repeated, such that it is less influential in terms of cultural transmission.

Innovation and creativity have been used interchangeably in the literature. For example, Lemmetty et al. (2021) contended that creativity includes two elements: originality and effectiveness. "The first criterion refers to the novelty and uniqueness of the creative product. The latter criterion pertains to the product's value and usability" (p. 2). Yet researchers often do make a distinction between creativity (i.e., exploring and generating ideas) and innovation (i.e., championing and implementing ideas) (De Jong & Den Hartog, 2010). Other researchers challenged the notion of alternative uses for assumed notions. They suggested that creativity underpins innovation, namely, innovation builds on the foundation of creative ideas (Argabright et al., 2012).

Hence, innovation appears to differ from creativity in that it also includes the strategic implementation of creative ideas. Creative individuals will more frequently express new ideas or multidimensional solutions to poorly structured problems, whereas innovative individuals also act to bring about a change (Etikariena, 2020). Anderson et al. (2014) viewed the innovation process as multilevel: "The creativity stage of this process refers to idea generation, and innovation to the subsequent stage of implementing ideas toward better procedures, practices, or products" (p. 1298).

In the context of higher education, innovation can be conceptualized in terms of the types of behavior students engage in to improve their learning or vocational processes. Researchers (e.g., Ness, 2021) underscored the importance of cultivating students' innovative skills during their studies before they enter the work market to better prepare them to deal with contemporary demands in the world of work and to cope with the requirements of their higher education learning environment.

Becker et al. (2018) emphasized the importance of stimulating students' innovation skills. Students should be encouraged to solve pressing challenges in order to shape their future. In this sense, higher education institutions are "incubators of inventions and developments" (p. 6). Thus, they should nurture a culture of entrepreneurial thinking through pedagogical practices such as project-based learning to create real-world experiences for learners. Higher education institutions should utilize active learning in which learners are perceived as partners in the process of knowledge creation: "Students do not have to wait until graduation to change the world" (p. 6).

In the context of healthcare studies, Lee and Lee (2021) asserted that in the aftermath of the COVID-19 pandemic, numerous organizations worldwide have experienced disruptions in production and logistic as a result of instability in their global supply chains. These disruptions have prompted many businesses to prioritize the creation of supply chains that are "less risky," albeit potentially "less efficient." The healthcare industry is among the sectors affected by these changes. In the digital age, healthcare providers and hospitals are actively seeking to foster innovation in the form of contactless services and operational processes, thereby improving productivity and organizational agility. This has been made possible by applying advanced information and communication technologies (ICTs), including artificial intelligence (AI), the Internet of Things (IoT), big data, 3D printing, virtual and augmented reality (VR/AR), smart sensors, robots, drones, and other similar technologies, which have been instrumental in implementing a range of contactless services.

Yet, even though the importance of cultivating innovation among students in higher education has been recognized, this topic has been inadequately addressed in the literature (Aboobaker & Zakkariya, 2019; Etikariena, 2020). Indeed, because higher education institutions continue to rely on traditional teacher-center paradigms, opportunities for advancing innovation skills are not being taken advantage of (Becker et al., 2018). Cramond and Fairweather (2013) voiced a similar criticism. They linked economic prosperity to a nation's creativity and strongly encouraged educators to nurture their students' creativity and innovation. At the same time, they pointed out that educators often "feel overwhelmed by the prospect of fitting one more thing into their already standards-crowded curriculum" (p. 245) and therefore do not attend to their student's social and emotional needs nor do they nurture creativity and innovation. The authors suggested FPS as a program that can be honed through existing courses, thus providing academic content while also enriching innovative thinking.

Future Problem Solving in Higher Education

The potential for engendering creativity and innovation skills inherent in Future Problem Solving (FPS) programs has been widely acknowledged, yet the environment for using such programs and identifying their benefits for higher education students is somewhat opaque, specifically in the case of future health managers. Nonetheless, several researchers have recently illustrated the benefit of FPS programs for higher education students. For example, in a quasi-experimental study, Alt et al. (2023) employed an FPS program in two study tracks: peace education and teacher training. Their main objective was to assess students' perceived awareness of future problem-solving, creativity and innovative behavior before and after program implementation. Another aim was to evaluate the potential links between the three variables. Three measurements were used to collect data from 432 students: *Awareness of Future Problems* scale*; Short Scale of Creative Self-SSCS;* and *Innovative Behavior* scale. The findings showed that by the end of the FPS program, the participants' awareness of future problems, their belief in their ability to produce creative ideas and their perceived innovative behavior had increased relative to program onset. The findings for the control group were not significant. The empirical model pointed to the mediating role of perceived creativity in linking awareness of future problems to students' perceived innovative behavior.

In the context of health management, Alt et al. (2022) examined an online FPS program conducted among 113 Israeli undergraduate students enrolled in a Management of Health Service Organizations course of study to determine what the program contributed to the students' eHealth literacy identity. The 62 participants in the research group received frequent weekly guidance that centered on enhancing their eHealth literacy skills, whereas the participants in the control group received minimal guidance from the lecturer. Data were gathered from both groups twice: pre- and post-program implementation. Only the research group exhibited significant increases in their perceived level of eHealth literacy skills between the two data collection points. This study shows that frequent and personalized guidance is needed to enhance skills in online educational environments. Educators must recognize the role of the instructor as a facilitator of learning and design successful scaffolding strategies to nurture students' lifelong learning skills during distance learning.

In the next section, we describe how an FPS program was implemented, step-by-step, in an online healthcare management course during the COVID-19 pandemic. The students were third-year undergraduates enrolled in healthcare systems management degree programs. First, we describe the phases of the intervention. Then we provide an example to illustrate the experience of the participating students. Finally, we analyze the students' reflections on their experience during the program.

Applying a Future Problem Solving Program in Healthcare Management Education

Eighty students were enrolled in a three-month FPS program that entailed the following six steps:

Step 1. In this phase, participants addressed a hypothetical scenario where a prolonged pandemic prevents face-to-face medical consultations, as outlined in the problem statement. They were informed about the ongoing COVID-19 pandemic with rising morbidity rates and no effective vaccine for new variants. This led to a strained health system with shortages of staff and medications, necessitating the shift to online patient consultations and remote hospitalizations. The challenge involved adapting to deliver diagnoses and treatments from a distance, with hospital visits limited to extreme cases only.

After being introduced to a broad challenge, students were grouped into teams of four to identify specific problems resulting from the scenario of prolonged lack of face-to-face medical interactions. They focused on impacts concerning patient-doctor relationships, service quality, ethics, and patient rights. Key issues included technological glitches, communication barriers, diagnostic limitations, patient cooperation difficulties, physicians' challenges with digital platforms, older adults' struggles with technology, and the erosion of personal connections in healthcare. These considerations highlighted the complexities of delivering remote medical services. In this step each group had to engage in preliminary research to understand the challenge and its related problems (Cramond, 2009). The groups considered such issues as varying levels of digital abilities in different population groups, the high cost of adapting the system, difficulties and opposition on the part of doctors and medical staff in adapting to the change, problems establishing intimate contact with medical staff and other issues.

Step 2. Each group selected one problem related to the specific challenge and formulated it as a question. For example: How can we solve the problem of access to online medical services among older adults or other population groups with limited digital skills? How can intimacy and trust between caregiver and patient be improved during online medical appointments?

Step 3. During this step, each group generated four solutions to the problem formulated in Step 2. They then held a brainstorming session during which they were instructed to imagine any solution that came to mind, regardless of its rationale or feasibility. To formulate their solutions, the groups accessed more information by reading materials related to the course content.

Step 4. In this step, the participants devised criteria for evaluating their proposed solutions. After small group discussions, each group created a Google Doc to which they could upload five ideal criteria. With the help of the students' suggestions, the lecturer then selected the five most appropriate assessment criteria. The criteria for assessing the solutions included the following: creative, easy to adapt, applicable, inexpensive in terms of manpower and funds, safe, has a long-term effect, does not require complicated technology, contributes to society as a whole.

Step 5. Each group evaluated their four solutions according to the criteria using a grid on which they indicated the value of each criterion on a Likert-type scale ranging from 1 = *not at all* to 6 = *absolutely*.

Step 6. Each group formulated an action plan to implement their chosen solution, outlining the steps needed, potential facilitators and detractors, and strategies for overcoming objections. The students presented their plans in a plenary session using online platforms like Thinglink. Proposed solutions included developing biometric security for medical confidentiality, establishing safe zones for online consultations, creating support systems for older adults to enhance their medical and digital literacy, and developing tools for remote diagnosis and treatment. In the following section we describe the output of this FPS program together with the students' reflections on their experience throughout the process. We provide the example as it was submitted by the group of students, without any modification or input from the lecturer. Note that this example does not necessarily constitute a realistic analysis of the potential consequences with respect to funding, feasibility or other relevant factors, but rather serves as a practice exercise for the students. The first step (introducing a future broad challenge and breaking it down into a number of problems) was executed in the form of an integrative discussion in which all the students in the group participated.

The Selected Problem: Manual Therapy

The group identified challenges related to the shift to online treatment during the COVID-19 pandemic, especially in scenarios requiring manual therapy. These cases involve essential physical contact for diagnosis or treatment, such as physiotherapy or rehabilitation after trauma. Treatments are tailored to each patient's physical, cognitive, and mental condition, requiring physiotherapists to assess various physical capabilities like range of motion and balance to make a diagnosis. In physiotherapy, direct physical contact is crucial and cannot be replicated remotely. If treatment is administered improperly or by unqualified individuals like friends or family, it could lead to rehabilitation setbacks or irreversible injuries.

The rising number of cases and increasing overload on hospitals and healthcare systems during the COVID-19 pandemic generated the need for digital treatment. Nevertheless, digital treatment often fails to provide patients the optimal treatment they need, raising questions such as the following: Can alternative forms of digital treatment be provided? Are other channels available for digital treatment?

The students noted that transitioning to long-distance medical treatment raises ideological and ethical concerns, particularly when treatments like manual therapy, which requires physical contact, are involved. Ethically, it's problematic if only those with access to necessary resources receive treatment, while others entitled to care under government health insurance do not, leading to inequality in healthcare provision.

Proposed Solutions to the Problem

The group proposed four solutions to the chosen problem.

Use of technology. To manage treatment demand and staff shortages, technology like sensor-based systems and mobile apps can facilitate remote rehabilitation. This allows caregivers to focus on in-person care for critical cases, while others receive guidance through devices such as smartphones and computers. Modern technology enables healthcare workers to check patients while they perform intensive, repetitive and challenging exercises. In most cases, patients can also receive ongoing digital feedback through systems that can report their achievements and progress during the rehabilitation program. Digital physiotherapy technologies have recently been developed that eliminate the need for a physiotherapist to administer treatment directly. Using these new technologies, patients can consult with physiotherapists on a forum via an application designed to provide accessible physiotherapy at home. The application can identify and analyze patient movements and offer corrections and instruction in real time so that patients can exercise independently.

Group Therapy. In cases where treatment does not have to be administered in the patient's bed, group therapy can be conducted in an open space for patients with similar needs and levels of difficulty. Group treatment, particularly in open spaces, offers a number of advantages. Institutions can more easily provide this type of treatment. It also saves money since a single healthcare worker with expertise can treat many patients simultaneously.

Group therapy offers a solution by being conducted outdoors, which frees up indoor treatment spaces for pandemic-related needs. It can also enhance patient recovery by providing a supportive environment where individuals see others with similar conditions making progress. This setting fosters mutual support, shared problem-solving, and feedback from both therapists and peers, encouraging patients to exert more effort and overcome challenges.

Hybrid Treatment. The approach combines home-based individual treatment with online long-distance care. Treatment at home allows therapists to address daily challenges in a familiar setting and advise family members on supporting the patient's exercises and home safety. Long-distance care provides continuous support when clinic visits are unfeasible and access to specialists in other regions. This blend of direct and online treatment enables more frequent sessions through telemedicine, reducing caregiver overload.

Treatment using Robots. The medical device market has been offering robots for use in telemedicine for some time. Such solutions must comply with the ethical laws governing the use of robotics. Robots are already performing surgical procedures without the presence of a surgeon, thus alleviating the need for contact between doctor and patient. Remote robotic operations are expanding to include other areas. Temi, a robot developed by Robotemi, an Israeli robotics company, is capable of conducting a series of medical examinations and administering medication at a relatively low cost. Robots operate using artificial intelligence; hence, their areas of treatment are constantly developing. Humanoid robots are capable of helping patients undergoing rehabilitation perform various exercises. The success of this type of rehabilitation depends on creating a trusting relationship between patient and robot.

The group evaluated each of these proposed solutions, as outlined in Steps 4 and 5. The group then selected a solution and constructed a plan for implementing it according to the final step of the intervention program.

The Selected Solution

The solution that received the most points was the use of robots for manual therapy.

Stages for Implementing the Solution

1. Developing or purchasing robots that can help patients with physiotherapy exercises, observe and monitor their progress, offer feedback and record the results in patients' medical files for examination by medical personnel. In addition, robots must include a mechanism for building trust between patient and robot.
2. Integrating the robots in medical centers and instructing caregivers on how to use the technology; teaching the medical staff how to program the robot with exercises, how to read the data output by the robot and how to instruct patients to use the robot.
3. Adapting the robot to the patient's needs: After conducting an in-person intake with the patient, the therapist must devise an individual treatment program based on the patient's condition. After that, an engineer will program the robot accordingly.
4. Pairing the robot with the patient: The therapist brings the robot to the patient's home and teaches the patient how to use it in accordance with the exercise program.
5. Adaptation period and building trust between patient and robot: The objective of this period is to increase trust between patient and robot. The patient must learn to understand that interacting with the robot is safe and that the robot's actions will enable the treatment to progress. The robot must be programmed according to the patient's physical limitations and language and must be taught to interpret the patient's mental condition according to physiological indexes.
6. Checking: After a predefined treatment period, the physiotherapist will assess the robot's output reports following each treatment and make changes accordingly.

Challenges and Opportunities

The challenge outlined here describes a situation in which physiotherapists cannot provide a direct face-to-face solution for their patients. The use of robots does not require personal contact, thus relieving the overload at medical centers. Moreover, the solution facilitates optimal long-distance treatment without exposing therapists or patients to COVID-19. The quality of treatment is not compromised since the robot is programmed according to the patient's needs.

Implementing this solution successfully requires contacting medical centers and the Ministry of Health's Medical and Technology Departments and explaining the solution's financial advantages and long-term benefits. In addition, the solution must be presented at conventions dedicated to medical technology and demonstrated at exhibits.

Opposition and Solutions

It is necessary to map where opposition is liable to arise in order to alleviate it. A survey we conducted on this issue revealed three main groups likely to express opposition to the proposed solution: the patients themselves, the physiotherapists and the insurance companies.

1. **Opposition from Patients**
   A. Patients with technophobia—Patients with technophobia may be unwilling to trust a robot as a medical assistant because they have doubts about its use and the reliability of its treatment. They may prefer to wait for an in-person meeting with a healthcare worker such as a physiotherapist rather than operate a technological device.
   B. Fear of hackers attacking the robot—Patients may fear that hackers could attack the robot, alter their treatment program, cause them harm or even access their medical information stored in the robot's computer and disseminate their private information.
   C. Patients who are resistant to deviations from traditional treatment—Patients may be hesitant to receive treatment from a robot. These include elderly patients who are not used to technological devices, are resistant to change or are accustomed to a permanent caregiver. They may feel that the robot cannot be trusted and may be unwilling to deviate from familiar traditional treatment.

To counter patient opposition to this form of treatment, we plan to produce films to increase patient awareness about the use and advantages of robots. We will also conduct workshops to introduce patients to the robots through practice sessions with the robot in the presence of their physiotherapist. Patients will also receive an explanation about the importance of treatment continuity and the dangers of discontinuing treatment for a lengthy period of time. Patients who are anxious about hackers will be assured that the robots are protected by an anti-hacking mechanism in order to alleviate their level of anxiety.

2. **Opposition from Therapists**

   A. Therapists who fear changes and are anxious about assimilating new technology may be opposed to the use of robots because they question the reliability of the data output by the robot after the treatment. They may also be afraid that the process of inputting patient data and programming the patient's exercises into the robot will be too complex and complicated for them. They may also fear they will not be able to install the exercise program properly or will mistakenly upload data liable to harm the patient.
   B. Medical students may fear that robots will begin to perform most treatments, so that by the time they complete their studies patients will prefer to receive treatment from a robot. They realize that robots will enable their patients to be treated at home at their own convenience rather than traveling to a clinic. Hence, they may be afraid that the demand for their profession will decrease, hindering their professional future for which they worked extremely hard.

Countering therapists' opposition will require working with the organizations and managers of healthcare clinics to convince therapists of the advantages of this type of treatment, including formulating a collective agreement that will ensure therapists' continued employment. The budget for this agreement will be deducted from the Ministry of Tourism, which has become inactive during the pandemic. We will provide explanations for therapists who are anxious about such changes to familiarize them with the use of robots and explain their advantages and benefits in the current situation.

3. **Opposition from Insurance Companies**

Insurance companies are liable to oppose this type of treatment because of its cost. They will have to pay technicians to maintain and repair the robots, transport the robots from one patient to another and remove them from the homes of patients who no longer require treatment.

Insurance companies who oppose this solution will have to be convinced by being informed of the financial benefits of using robots.

The group was also asked to describe why one of their proposed solutions was rejected. The proposed solution they chose to discuss was the use of modern technologies for checking and monitoring patients as they perform exercises while receiving long-distance directions from a physiotherapist via sensory systems and applications on digital devices such as a computer, tablet, or smartphone. The group did not choose this solution because it is not suitable to the entire population. Indeed, such a solution would be inaccessible to people who do not believe in using digital devices, have no Internet access in their homes or have difficulty using such devices. Because these people would not be able to receive online treatment, the group rejected this solution.

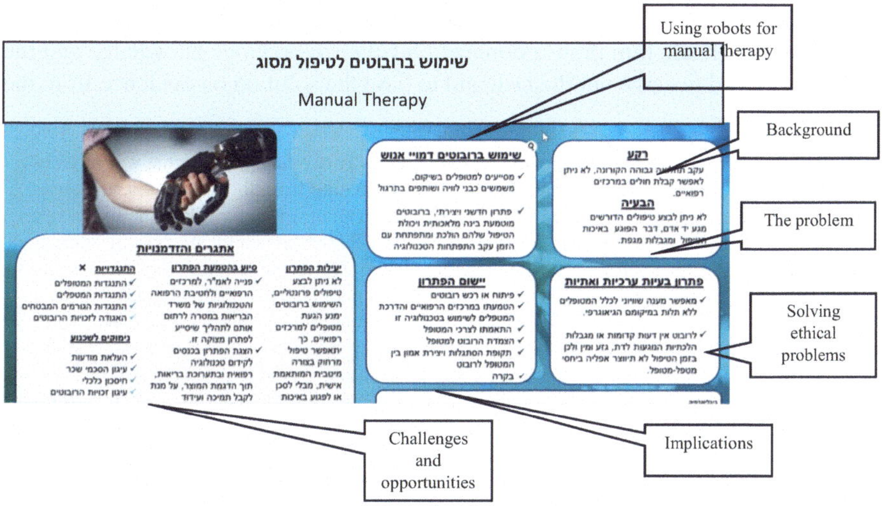

Fig. 5.1 A screenshot from the action plan presentation

The students presented their action plan using a narrated digital poster that illustrated the main points of the plan and provided explanations about its implementation, as shown in Fig. 5.1.

Students' Reflections

The students were asked to write a reflective journal throughout the activity to record their thoughts and feelings. The following sections offer a thematic analysis of the journals written by four group members. The journals revealed four categories: perceived innovation and creativity, multidirectional observation, assessment of ethical aspects and challenges encountered during the activity.

Perceived Innovation and Creativity

The students who participated in the activity reported that the tasks required them to think as a group about future problems elicited by the described challenge. Each member of the group proposed ideas for defining the problem concisely and reached a joint decision that the problem of accessibility of long-distance treatment was relevant in situations in which manual therapy was required. According to the group, "We chose a problem that required more creativity and thinking." Adam explained that the instructions to think of several solutions presented a challenge: "We were forced to think of several solutions and not just one or two. We looked for a creative and innovative solution while using flexible, out-of-the-box thinking." Adam stressed that the process made him draw a connection between previous knowledge and the thinking required to carry out the task and to base the solution on evidence from the study materials.

> The assignment required me to think in an innovative way over and above what was already obvious in order to find a solution to the problems emerging from the case study (the challenge). Despite the difficulty in finding a creative innovative solution, I liked the task a lot. It required me to think in a different way. In a previous lesson on healthcare systems abroad we learned about the healthcare system in Japan, where robots were being used for various purposes such as alleviating loneliness among elderly people. This made me think about a solution that involved long-distance treatment using robots. At first not everyone in the group agreed that robots could solve the problem. Some group members felt this was impossible. We searched for articles about robots in healthcare and discovered that a robot had recently been invented that could solve the problem. That article proved to all members of the group that our solution was possible, and this was the solution we presented on our poster.

Edna also noted that the task enabled her to assess the current reality more intensely in order to find solutions to the problem.

> During the search for the solution I began to understand that we didn't have to reinvent the wheel (in this case, the robot). When you are coping with a current or future problem, you have to look around and ask: "What is out there? What solutions already exist?" The solution might be spearhead technology or an older product. You have to examine it and examine how you can make adaptations, changes or combinations according to what is needed to solve the problem.

Multidirectional Observation

Inbal described the advantages of the approach for developing creativity and innovation. She focused on the fact that the approach "forces the participants to examine numerous viewpoints":

> I think that the advantage of this learning approach for me as a student was that this type of work forced me to analyze and think differently in order to fulfill the various requirements of the assignment. This approach helped me think about the future problem in the case study from a different standpoint. I had to find a creative and innovative solution to the problems emerging from the article. The process helped me assess the situation from a different perspective. If at the beginning of the semester I thought that the number of solutions to this problem was relatively limited, I came to realize that there were many possible solutions.

The students in the group emphasized the need to work as a group to find a solution. Edna emphasized the importance of diversity in the group that contributed to creative thinking:

> The problem had to be solved by a group of people and not by one person. The group should preferably be heterogeneous and made up of people of both genders from different social and academic backgrounds. A mixed group will generate varied ways of thinking and different viewpoints to overcome the challenge. This will lessen the chances of intellectual stagnation and becoming locked on one particular issue. Cooperation contributes to finding non-conventional directions of thinking.

Assessing Ethical Aspects

One of the criteria for evaluating the quality of the solution revolved around ethics. The students were asked to assess the solution while examining the repercussions of its implementation upon humanity. Inbal described how the group members were exposed to less desirable aspects of using robots while they searched for a solution, among them financial harm to weak population groups. She pointed to the lack of up-to-date legislation and feared that the work of experts would become superfluous as a result of integrating robots in this profession.

> While we were writing up the solutions, I wondered if we needed to ask modern philosophers to write a working paper discussing this topic. It seems that most considerations of this issue are influenced by science fiction in one way or another. I found myself thinking about this even after we submitted the poster.

Challenges During the Activity

The main difficulties raised by members of the group fell into two categories. The first was technological difficulties. For example, Liat described the challenges of presenting the action plan by means of a digital poster:

> I learned to use two new computer programs - Thinglink and Pictochart – while making the poster. I enjoyed learning and using them. One of the difficulties in building the poster was formulating the contents in a focused concise manner while presenting all the relevant information we wanted to show. We wanted to display the poster in an innovative way that would be interesting. This required us to be creative.

Another interesting difficulty the group members described pertained to the waning of the COVID-19 pandemic and the apparent disappearance of the challenges it brought. As the semester progressed, the challenge became more obscure and less relevant. The students seemed to have difficulty conceptualizing something that no longer existed. Inbal explained:

> The main obstacle was the transition to an imaginary world. It became more difficult to deal with a problem that no longer existed, and the group found it hard to engage in a game of "let's pretend." In my opinion, proposing the solution did not benefit us directly. Nevertheless, we benefitted from the understanding that we needed to look at challenges from different points of view.

Discussion

In this chapter we demonstrated how a six-step FPS program can be employed in health management courses. The participants were asked to address a future challenge and suggest practical solutions. The proposed FPS program encouraged participants to generate new and multiple solutions to poorly structured problems and to identify unknown factors and seek clarity by creating links among remotely associated issues (Ritter & Ferguson, 2017). The students also acknowledged that the program promoted their creativity, thus pointing to the benefits of student awareness of social challenges and their perceived ability to offer solutions, evaluate solution quality and devise an action plan to implement their creative ideas (Treffinger et al., 2021). Corroboration for this can be found in a study by Masek and Yamin (2010), who maintained that problem-based learning appears to offer potential in fostering student creativity by developing specific components of creativity, such as domain- and creative-relevant sets of skills.

Moreover, the example cited here suggests that innovative behavior can be prompted by students' enhanced awareness of future social problems and their solutions, in line with the premise of Joachim et al. (2020) that unconstrained and futuristic thinking is a critical mindset in the pursuit of innovation. FPS programs require skills that are directed beyond that which is immediately known and familiar and that are consistent with contemporary views that learning is a process of constructing or reconstructing knowledge to attend to a new situation. Situations introduced by FPS programs require innovative thinking because existing models or solution strategies are unavailable or unproductive (Alt & Raichel, 2018).

Our experience also points to the benefits of using FPS to promote awareness of social challenges among health care management students and to foster their ability to offer solutions, evaluate solution quality and devise an action plan for solution implementation. Indeed, previous investigations into FPS (Alt et al., 2023) underscored its benefits for developing problem-solving skills, raising awareness of future problems and taking responsibility for solving problems. Hence, practicing and learning to deal with possible future challenges by suggesting logical and creative solutions and devising plans to appropriately cope may motivate students to delve more deeply into challenging situations in the present.

We advocate programs that develop future thinking about social and medical issues in order to promote innovation and creativity among healthcare management students. The practice proposed in this study may be beneficial in enhancing these lifelong learning skills in that it not only introduces problems that require learners to recall previously learned knowledge in a new situation but also spurs learners to imagine possible solutions and to rethink key ideas, customs and even values in order to change and adapt to changing circumstances. FPS programs kindle students' adaptability by leading them to recognize the cognitive power to change their environments as they encounter novel situations.

We therefore recommend integrating the FPS technique into healthcare education curricula by posing poorly structured problems with no clear starting points or goals and multiple potential solutions. Learners should be exposed to incongruence between the given and desired situation and should acknowledge that bridging this gap requires solutions that are not readily at hand. Indeed, such a situation requires finding unconventional solutions to the problem, offering the potential to improve learners' problem-solving ability, instigate their belief in the centrality of their own creativity in their overall self-description and promote the innovative abilities they need for learning and for their future professional careers.

References

Aboobaker, N., & Zakkariya, K. A. (2019). Influence of digital learning orientation and readiness for change on innovative work behaviour: Reflections from the higher education sector. *International Journal of Educational Management, 35*(5), 1030–1047. https://doi.org/10.1108/DLO-08-2019-0191

Alt, D., & Raichel, N. (2018). *Lifelong citizenship: Lifelong learning as a lever for moral and democratic values*. Brill and Sense Publishers. https://doi.org/10.1163/9789463512398

Alt, D., Naamati-Schneider, L., & Meirovich, A. (2022). Future problem-solving practiced during Covid-19: Implications for health management students' e-Health literacy identity. *Frontiers in Psychology*. https://doi.org/10.3389/fpsyg.2022.829243

Alt, D., Kapshuk, Y., & Dekel, H. (2023). Promoting perceived creativity and innovative behavior: Benefits of future problem-solving programs for higher education students. *Thinking Skills and Creativity, 47*. https://doi.org/10.1016/j.tsc.2022.101201

Alzahrani, A. A., Al-Dhaimat, Y., & Shahin, A. (2020). The effectiveness of future problem-solving program (FPSP) in developing creative thinking skills among gifted students: Experimental study. *Journal of Education and Practice, 11*, 154–171. https://doi.org/10.5296/ijld.v9i4.15893

Anderson, N., Potocnik, K., & Zhou, J. (2014). Innovation and creativity in organizations: A state-of-the-science review, prospective commentary, and guiding framework. *Journal of Management, 40*(5), 1–37. https://doi.org/10.1177/0149206314527128

Argabright, K., McGuire, J., & King, J. (2012). Extension through a new lens: Creativity and innovation now and for the future. *Journal of Extension, 50*(2), article 39. https://doi.org/10.34068/joe.50.02.39

Azevedo, I., de Fátima Morais, M., & Martins, F. (2019). The future problem-solving program international: An intervention to promote creative skills in Portuguese adolescents. *The Journal of Creative Behavior, 53*(3), 263–273. https://doi.org/10.1002/jocb.175

Azevedo, I., Morais, M. D. F., Martins, F., & Cramond, B. (2016). *The future problem solving program international (FPSPI): A challenge for creative citizens*. Kie Conference Publishing. Retrieved from https://repositorium.sdum.uminho.pt/handle/1822/42299

Becker, S. A., Brown, M., Dahlstrom, E., Davis, A., DePaul, K., Diaz, V., & Pomerantz, J. (2018). NMC horizon report: 2018 higher education edition. *Educause*.

Carr, K., Kendal, R. L., & Flynn, E. G. (2016). Eureka! What is innovation, how does it develop, and who does it? *Child Development, 87*(5), 1505–1519. https://doi.org/10.1111/cdev.12549

Cramond, B. L. (2009). Future problem solving in gifted education. In L. V. Shavinina (Ed.), *International handbook on giftedness* (pp. 1143–1156). Springer.

Cramond, B. L., & Fairweather, E. C. (2013). Future problem solving as education for innovation. In L. V. Shavinina (Ed.), *The Routledge international handbook of innovation education* (pp. 245–256). Routledge.

Czerwonka, M., & Karwowski, M. (2018). The order matters: Asking about creative activity calibrates creative self-concept. *Creativity Research Journal, 30*, 179–186. https://doi.org/10.1080/10400419.2018.1446499

De Jong, J., & Den Hartog, D. (2010). Measuring innovative work behaviour. *Creativity and Innovation Management, 19*(1), 23–36. https://doi.org/10.1111/j.1467-8691.2010.00547.x

Dochy, F., & Segers, M. (2018). *Creating impact through future learning: The high impact learning that lasts (HILL) model*. Routledge.

Etikariena, A. (2020). Encouraging innovative work behavior among college students through quality education to succeed the SDGs. In *E3S Web of Conferences* (Vol. 211). EDP Sciences. https://doi.org/10.1051/e3sconf/202021101016

Joachim, G., Schulenkorf, N., Schlenker, K., & Frawley, S. (2020). Design thinking and sport for development: Enhancing organizational innovation. *Managing Sport and Leisure, 25*(3), 175–202. https://doi.org/10.1080/23750472.2019.1611471

Karwowski, M., & Barbot, B. (2016). Creative self-beliefs: Their nature, development, and correlates. In J. C. Kaufman & J. Baer (Eds.), *Cambridge companion to reason and development* (pp. 302–326). Cambridge University Press.

Kashani-Vahid, L., Afrooz, G., Shokoohi-Yekta, M., Kharrazi, K., & Ghobari, B. (2017). Can a creative interpersonal problem solving program improve creative thinking in gifted elementary students? *Thinking Skills and Creativity, 24*, 175–185. https://doi.org/10.1016/j.tsc.2017.02.011

Lauring, J., & Selmer, J. (2013). Self-initiated expatriates in the private versus the public sector: Creativity and work outcomes. *International Journal of Public Administration, 36*(9), 649–658. https://doi.org/10.1080/01900692.2013.791310

Lee, S. M., & Lee, D. (2021). Opportunities and challenges for contactless healthcare services in the post-COVID-19 era. *Technological Forecasting and Social Change, 167*, 120712. https://doi.org/10.1016/j.techfore.2021.120712

Lemmetty, S., Glăveanu, V. P., Forsman, P., & Collin, K. (2021). Introduction: Creativity and learning as sociocultural and intertwined phenomena. In *Creativity and learning* (pp. 1–24). Palgrave Macmillan. https://doi.org/10.1007/978-3-030-77066-2_12

Luu, T. T., Rowley, C., Dinh, C. K., Qian, D., & Le, H. Q. (2019). Team creativity in public healthcare organizations: The roles of charismatic leadership, team job crafting, and collective public service motivation. *Public Performance & Management Review, 42*(6), 1448–1480. https://doi.org/10.1080/15309576.2019.1595067

Main, L. F., Delcourt, M. A., & Treffinger, D. J. (2019). Effects of group training in problem-solving style on future problem-solving performance. *The Journal of Creative Behavior, 53*(3), 274–285. https://doi.org/10.1002/jocb.176

Masek, A., & Yamin, S. (2010). Fostering creativity from the constructivist perspectives: A literature review. In *Proceeding of the 3rd Regional Conference on Engineering Education & Research in Higher Education*. School of Professional and Continuing Education (UTMspace), Universiti Teknologi Malaysia.

Mumford, M., Hunter, S., & Byrne, C. (2009). What is the fundamental? The role of cognition in creativity and innovation. *Industrial and Organizational Psychology, 2*, 353–356. https://doi.org/10.1111/j.1754-9434.2009.01158.x

Ness, I. J. (2021). Mind the gap: Creative knowledge processes within interdisciplinary groups in organizations and higher education. In S. Lemmetty, K. Collin, V. P. Glăveanu, & P. Forsman (Eds.), *Creativity and learning: Contexts, processes and support* (pp. 195–217). Palgrave Macmillan. https://doi.org/10.1007/978-3-030-77066-2_9

Pretz, J. E., & Nelson, D. (2017). Creativity is influenced by domain, creative self-efficacy, mindset, self-efficacy, and self-esteem. In M. Karwowski, & J. C. Kaufman (Eds.), *The creative self* (pp. 242–270). Academic Press. https://doi.org/10.1016/B978-0-12-809790-8.00009-1

Ritter, S. M., & Ferguson, S. (2017). Happy creativity: Listening to happy music facilitates divergent thinking. *PloS one, 12*(9). https://doi.org/10.1371/journal.pone.0182210

Runco, M. A., & Jaeger, G. J. (2012). The standard definition of creativity. *Creativity Research Journal, 24*, 92–96. https://doi.org/10.1080/10400419.2012.650092

Torrance, E. P., & Cramond, B. (2002). Needs of creativity programs, training, and research in the schools of the future. *Research in the Schools, 9*(2), 5–14. https://doi.org/10.4236/jss.2015.36010

Torrance, E. P., & Torrance, J. P. (1978). Developing creativity instruction materials according to the Osborn-Parnes creative problem solving model. *Creative Child and Adult Quarterly, 3*, 80–90.

Treffinger, D. J., Solomon, M., & Woythal, D. (2012). Four decades of creative vision: Insights from an evaluation of the future problem solving program international (FPSPI). *Journal of Creative Behavior, 46*, 209–219. https://doi.org/10.1002/jocb.14

Treffinger, D. J., Schoonover, P. F., & Selby, E. C. (2021). *Educating for creativity & innovation: A comprehensive guide for research-based practice*. Routledge.

Vijayaratnam, P. (2012). Developing higher order thinking skills and team commitment via group problem solving: A bridge to the real world. *Procedia-Social and Behavioral Sciences, 66*, 53–63. https://doi.org/10.1016/j.sbspro.2012.11.247

Zhou, Z., & Verburg, R. (2020). Open for business: The impact of creative team environment and innovative behaviour in technology-based start-ups. *International Small Business Journal, 38*(4), 318–336. https://doi.org/10.1177/0266242619892793

Chapter 6
Digital Transformation: Building eHealth Literacy Skills Among Healthcare Managers

Abstract In an era marked by rapid digital transformation, building eHealth literacy skills among healthcare managers is vital. This chapter examines the integration of digital technologies in healthcare and their role in enhancing organizational performance and patient care. It focuses on developing eHealth literacy, defined as the ability to access, evaluate, and apply digital medical information. The chapter highlights an intervention program employing the Future Problem Solving (FPS) method, which significantly improved students' eHealth literacy skills, emphasizing the importance of innovative teaching methods in healthcare education. The chapter underscores the necessity of innovative educational approaches to equip healthcare professionals with essential digital skills, ensuring they can navigate and adapt to the evolving healthcare landscape

Introduction

In recent years, the healthcare system has had to cope with mounting changes on both the local and the global levels (Naamati Schneider, 2020, 2022; WHO, 2019). In the wake of the COVID-19 outbreak in December 2019, the rate of these changes accelerated dramatically. To respond to these changes, the healthcare system must take specific steps to help its workers on all levels acquire new skills that can facilitate their adaptation to these changes (Deshpande et al., 2023). During the last decade, as healthcare organizations attempted to adapt to these shifting environments, they began to embrace digital transformation. Indeed, increased use of digital technologies was among the substantial and far-reaching organizational changes necessitated by the new situation. This direction has served a variety of functions, such as enhancing business performance, improving customer experience, streamlining organizational processes, and implementing innovative business models (Naamati-Schneider, 2023; Naamati-Schneider & Salvatore, 2022, 2023; Topol, 2012).

By embracing digital transformation during the COVID-19 pandemic, healthcare organizations have been able to expand their activity and retain their customers.

L. Naamati-Schneider and D. Alt, *Technology and Competency-Oriented Learning*,
https://doi.org/10.1007/978-981-97-5771-8_6

Furthermore, this transformation generated digitally based sources of income. Collaborations with startups, biotech companies, and other technological companies provided immediate solutions to newly emerging problems. These solutions included remote medical services, digital healthcare, remote data analysis, distant patient monitoring, and touch-free treatment. They also involved cutting edge robotics and innovative respiratory devices, patient-adjusted healthcare, telemedicine, digitalized customer services, computerized management of patient records, and digitally based care continuity (Kraus et al., 2021; Marques & Ferreira, 2020; Naamati-Schneider & Zaks, 2022; Schwab, 2017).

This digital transformation has also changed the relationship between patients and healthcare providers and has played a key role in re-orienting healthcare services toward a more patient-focused approach. Consequently, the role of the physician shifted, and the accessibility of services improved. Reflecting these new directions, internet-based platforms (e.g., social media, forums, blogs, medical consultation websites, and AI-based applications) have become arenas for collecting and sharing medical information (Jarva et al., 2023; Maeda & Socha-Dietrich, 2021).

To adjust to these changes, the healthcare system must help its workers acquire the skills needed to adapt. These may include various communication and learning capacities such as problem-solving abilities and digital literacy (Khan et al., 2022; Veikkolainen et al., 2023). Such lifelong learning skills have become vital for healthcare professionals. Therefore, higher education in the field of healthcare must include these skills in its training programs, a goal that can be achieved via innovative teaching methods (Berkhout et al., 2018).

Digital literacy is considered a key component in the set of twenty-first century tools and skills, especially in light of the currently accelerating digital transformation worldwide (Khan et al., 2022). Online health literacy, or eHealth literacy, is defined as the capacity to access, evaluate, and apply medical information from digital sources. Indeed, eHealth literacy is taking root and is now recognized as an important element in health literacy in general and a crucial ability for workers and managers in the field (Alt et al., 2022).

In this chapter we examine the development and assimilation of health literacy skills in healthcare organizations and among medical teams. We review projects designed to develop such skills and demonstrate these efforts by introducing a program intended to reinforce eHealth literacy skills among students majoring in healthcare systems management. The program employed the methodologies of future case study through the use of e-posters.

Health and eHealth Literacy Skills in an Everchanging Environment

The concept *literacy* has expanded over time. Initially, it was mainly used to describe the ability to read and write, to understand and work with numbers (numeracy), and to solve problems (Alt & Raichel, 2020; National Literacy Act, 1991). Today, however, literacy has broadened to encompass personal knowledge and potential in a range of areas, such as science, medicine, or finance, and now includes various skills. According to UNESCO (2018), digital literacy requires more than merely knowing how to operate a computer. It includes fundamental skills as well as living skills that apply to all aspects of modern life.

Similarly, the concept of *health literacy* has also been expanded in response to changes in the environment and the needs of the population. Today health literacy encompasses three levels: functional, interactive and evaluative (Nutbeam & McGill, 2019).

Functional health literacy, for example, refers to the ability to understand fact-based information related to medical risks and treatment options. This skill allows individuals to understand medical information that originates from well-established and reliable sources, such as medical brochures distributed at health centers. Both individuals and communities need to master this skill, which can improve the response to programs intended to promote public health. On the *interactive level*, medical literacy is reflected in the ability to interact with healthcare providers. This skill strengthens people's capacity to act independently and be self-motivated and confident in communicating and collaborating with medical practitioners. In terms of society, this skill exerts a major influence on social norms and communication between population groups.

Evaluative health literacy refers to the ability to evaluate and use existing medical information. Evaluative health literacy allows people to be critical of social and political processes that affect healthcare. On the individual level, evaluative health literacy contributes to people's commitment to social and economic challenges in healthcare, while on the community level it empowers social activities that promote healthcare (Walters et al., 2020). Through these three levels, medical literacy acquires meaning both for individuals and for society. As an example, understanding medical brochures contributes to individual health, but also carries social implications in terms of health promotion, public costs, and inequity in healthcare (Mehoudar, 2014).

Online eHealth Literacy

In recent years, the concept of online eHealth literacy has gained momentum. This concept is defined as the ability to search for, find, and understand health-related information retrieved from electronic sources, to evaluate its quality, and to rely on it when dealing with illness to optimize medical outcomes. eHealth literacy comprises various components of literacy.

Several studies have examined the link between the health and disease prevention characteristics of a particular population and the levels of medical and online medical literacy found in that group. Yang et al. (2017) showed that high levels of evaluative health literacy predicted dimensions of healthy lifestyle, such as health responsibility, wholesome nutrition, resilience to stress, and physical exercise. Other studies reinforced these findings. In Japan, for instance, Mitsutake et al. (2016) found that high levels of online health literacy correlated with a healthy diet and exercise. Similarly, Tennant et al. (2015) found that online medical literacy positively correlated with socioeconomic status, education, and frequency of technology use (Tennant et al., 2015). These studies and others employed various research methodologies commonly used for evaluating online medical literacy. One such measure is the Lily model, which tests basic literacy, health literacy, information literacy, media literacy, computer literacy, and science literacy. Another is the eHEALS (eHealth Literacy Scale) questionnaire, a self-report utterance-rating scale (Norman & Skinner, 2006).

Other studies showed that low levels of medical literacy in a population were tied to limited knowledge about health and illness, poor health, and higher rates of hospitalization relative to the population average (Diviani et al., 2015). Mullan et al. (2017) revealed a direct link between low health literacy and measures such as poor health, deficient understanding of medical conditions, unhealthy lifestyle, poor education, and low socioeconomic status among ethnically diverse adults (Mullan et al., 2017). Other researchers (e.g., Sørensen et al., 2015) demonstrated varying levels of health literacy among specific populations, such as older adults, people with low levels of education, minorities, people with limited access to resources, and people with low socioeconomic status.

These findings point to the practical implications of health literacy for public health. In addition, during the past decade the medical field has been inundated with information, with social media and other internet platforms offering the public easy access to reports whose reliability is often questionable. This situation underscores the importance of developing medical literacy skills to promote individual and community health (Deshpande et al., 2023; Paakkari & Okan, 2020; Mehoudar, 2014; Rueda-Medina et al., 2023).

Online eHealth Literacy Education

Research shows that educating the population and improving general and online medical literacy are highly important for disease prevention and treatment. These factors are also crucial for achieving cooperation in the relationship between patients and healthcare providers and for reducing inequity in health (Mehoudar, 2014). The consequences of the global COVID-19 pandemic highlighted the importance of this issue, when it became clear that a lack of medical education and insufficient health literacy had adverse effects on public health. Paakkari and Okan (2020) showed that population groups that were educated about health issues, including contagion, hygiene, and vaccination, exhibited better cooperation at a time when public response to health guidelines was crucial.

Digital developments, considered part of the fourth industrial revolution, affect not only the general population but professionals in the field as well (Schwab, 2017). For both patients and healthcare personnel, these changes necessitate substantial accessibility to digital information, generating a growing need for appropriate tools to process information and examine its reliability (Hemmo-Lotem & Shani, 2018; Schwab, 2017; Veikkolainen et al., 2023).

Furthermore, rapid technological changes play an important role in personalized medicine. Because personalized medicine is based on big data, physicians and patients alike must be able to understand and process these data. An additional development in the field of healthcare is the use of artificial intelligence (Hemmo-Lotem & Shani, 2018). These changes—some of which have already been instituted while others are projected—are expected to become part of the healthcare system in the near and more distant future. Hence, as individuals and healthcare professionals adapt to the shifting reality of the fourth industrial revolution and its effect on the world of medicine, their medical literacy must be improved (Mullan et al., 2017; Schwab, 2017). Indeed, improving these skills among healthcare professionals as well as the general public will have meaningful benefits, among them enhanced patient safety, disease prevention, and improved health. Improved medical literacy will also contribute to better relationships between patients and healthcare providers, increased social equity, and reduced resistance to change (Hemmo-Lotem et al., 2021).

The above survey leads to the conclusion that medical literacy skills should be developed among students in medical and healthcare management programs at the early stages of their training. Such education is critical for their future work in the field and their success in adapting to changing demands. Kaper et al. (2019) found that developing online medical literacy promotes self-management among both patients and healthcare professionals, leading to better care management as healthcare paradigms shift and the physicians' role changes. Furthermore, among healthcare providers, mastery of digital skills was found to be an effective tool for dealing with the fear, stress, and anxiety that are prevalent under conditions of onerous workloads and uncertainty, such as during the COVID-19 pandemic (Nguyen et al., 2020).

Enhancing eHealth Literacy via Educational Intervention Programs

The development of health literacy and online health literacy has been examined in specific population groups. For example, Nagler et al. (2013) conducted an intervention study at Harvard in communities marked by low socioeconomic status (59%

below the poverty line). The participants were offered workshops to develop their health literacy and promote their health, e.g., classes to teach people how to use computers and the internet, including how to search for health-related information. The study was conducted in three phases. In each phase, there were nine consecutive monthly training sessions conducted at community colleges in Boston. Addition to the training, participants were provided with computers, internet access and instructions for navigating the internet, and ongoing technical support. The researchers discovered numerous complexities during the intervention and reported inconclusive results.

Xie (2011) developed an intervention program for older adults, who were given two weeks of training in how to use websites to look for information. The participants reported positive attitudes toward the program and became more involved in their own medical treatment. Lopez and Grant (2012) described an intervention program targeting Hispanic people with diabetes in the United States. The program used a specialized software package called eNavigator, which was found to have the potential to improve the online health literacy of this population group.

Research (Stellefson et al., 2011) targeting student populations found that students felt comfortable using the internet to look up medical information. Nevertheless, an assessment of their eHealth literacy found it to be deficient. The researchers stressed that the reported gaps were especially problematic for students in the healthcare professions and recommended providing specialized training for this group focusing on using the internet for medical purposes. Other researchers also encouraged the development of such skills among students (Rueda-Medina et al., 2023).

Several studies examined the development of literacy skills through problem-solving methods. Frank and Castek (2017), for example, contended that advancing basic digital literacy skills is insufficient, stating that teachers should prepare their students to "skillfully use digital tools and develop a discovery and risk-taking mindset toward navigating online" (p. 66). Such efforts require developing digital problem-solving abilities rather than basic digital skills. These abilities include locating, evaluating, creating, and communicating information to solve poorly structured real-world problems in technology-rich environments (Quann, 2015).

Despite the scope of these studies, very few researchers have examined development of online literacy skills among students in healthcare professions. Furthermore, not much research has been dedicated to integrating problem-solving abilities while employing literacy skills. This is despite the fact that problem-solving skills are crucial for medical teams, as they must be capable of solving immediate problems in real-time situations and of synthesizing their personal knowledge when dealing with the challenges presented by a world that is constantly changing (El-Benny et al., 2021).

Future Problem-Solving Implemented During COVID-19: Implications for the eHealth Literacy Identity of Health Management Students

The authors of this book (Alt et al., 2022) conducted a study to examine an intervention program designed for undergraduate students in health systems management. The intervention program was based on implementation of an online Future Problem Solving (FPS) program in the field of health education.

Future Problem-Solving programs use complex, open-ended problems that are based on daily situations, relevant to the future, and rooted in social contexts. The problems are designed in the form of an inquisitive activity that calls upon students to devise creative solutions and encourages them to develop skills they can apply throughout their lives (Main et al., 2019). Fostering the ability to solve future problems has been the focus of numerous educational programs (Treffinger et al., 2021).

Future Problem-Solving Intervention Program

The aim of the intervention program was to enhance students' eHealth literacy identity using two levels of teacher guidance: minimal vs. frequent. Students in the research group (62) were provided regular weekly guidance that focused on enhancing their eHealth literacy skills. In contrast, students in the control group (51) received minimal guidance from the course instructor. In both groups, data were gathered twice: pre- and post-implementation of the program. The program comprised the following six sequential steps (Cramond, 2009; Torrance & Cramond, 2002): (1) identifying challenges in a future problematic situation; (2) selecting an underlying problem to be tackled based on the presented situation; (3) offering possible solutions to the selected problem without judgment; (4) creating and selecting criteria for evaluating the suggested solutions; (5) evaluating and ranking the possible solutions according to the selected criteria and choosing the optimal one; and (6) developing an action plan to demonstrate how the solution will work to solve the underlying problem (Cramond, 2009).

Different levels of teacher guidance were provided based on research demonstrating that teacher assistance is pivotal in online courses (Kim et al., 2014). Numerous studies (Alt & Naamati-Schneider, 2021, 2022; Garcia et al., 2018; Kebritchi et al., 2017) have shown that distance and online learning in higher education changed the role of teachers and the way students learn. Specific learning styles and skills are required for successful participation in online courses. Hence, instructors in such courses should identify learners who lack technical knowledge, time management skills, and other relevant abilities, and should provide specific assistance to these students.

To assess and measure students' perceived digital skills in using information technology for health, the researchers administered the eight-item eHEALS Scale (Norman & Skinner, 2006). Data were collected from both groups before and after program implementation. The findings showed significant differences only for the research group, with increased levels of eHealth literacy skills detected between the tests. Only the research group perceived that the FPS program had made a significant contribution to their eHealth literacy skill, whereas the results for the control group were not significant.

The researchers conducted an additional study among undergraduate students in their final year of studies in a healthcare systems management program. These students went through the same intervention program based on the FBL methodology. In addition, they employed digital tools to remotely create an E-poster. The students were further asked to contemplate their personal learning process during this activity and to submit a reflective journal in which they described their challenges and gains during the learning experience. To do so, participants were given reflective prompts (Tripto et al., 2016) such as: "Describe the main challenges and difficulties that emerged during the activity" or "Describe what worked well and what did not work well during the learning activity." This practice encouraged the students to document their thoughts during the activity and prompted them to think and write about their learning in a multidimensional way (Alt & Raichel, 2020; Zohar & Barzilai, 2013). The entries were typically eight to ten paragraphs long.

The students in the intervention program expanded their knowledge by locating sources on the internet and using the information they found to devise solutions to an important future problem. Then they evaluated the proposed solutions and documented their own learning. The study also employed the case study method, defined by Yin (2012) as an empirical investigation of a current phenomenon (the case) and its linkage to the real world. The case study method entails observations and data collection from human activity at a specific time and place, allowing the researcher to learn certain things about the processes under investigation. Similar to other qualitative study methods, here too the researcher identifies themes or categories emerging from the participants' words. When writing up the scientific report, the researcher serves as the participants' voice, such that every claim or generalization deriving from their words is established empirically through quotes (Guba & Lincoln, 2002).

Analysis of Reflective Journals Written by Students in the Intervention Program

In the current case study, the students' reflective journals were analyzed to examine the challenges and opportunities embedded in the suggested method for developing online eHealth literacy. Based on theory and analysis of the content of the journals, four categories emerged: (1) ability to search for and find material; (2) facilitation of information use; (3) development of critical literacy skills; and (4) contribution of task sequence.

Ability to Search for and Find Material

In this category, the students reported that they were challenged by the demand to engage in active learning, which diverged from their familiar learning patterns. Indeed, as Dana indicated, this learning style pushed them to develop a sense of competence in their ability to locate material relevant to their studies:

> My participation in the lessons of the course enriched my learning abilities and my perception of knowledge, unlike the learning experience of receiving knowledge passively. I was "forced" to leave my comfort zone and search for knowledge and materials in different and diverse ways, and I was successful!

Luna's reflective journal reflects the same sentiments:

> For the first time, in my third year of studies, I had a lot of difficulty finding solutions to a problem and determining how to write them up. On the other hand, I also experienced a sense of satisfaction in accessing and finding the material I needed to get results.

These descriptions of the search for material and the gradual acquisition of knowledge emphasize the nature of learning as a process. The students felt that rather than aiming for a final product, they went through a process of looking up information and reaching a solution—a process that turned out to be an integral part of the learning. Lina stated:

> During my years at college and in school or any other place of learning in general, I felt that what was most important was the final result and not the way it was achieved. Here you can see clearly that the way was most important.

Nevertheless, many of the participating students reported being challenged by the FBL methodology, which employed unfamiliar teaching patterns and forced them to cope with active learning while locating sources of information and using them to achieve the desired result. They indicated that this process was complex and entailed numerous difficulties, particularly the intense efforts required to complete the large number of tasks. Dani, for example, indicated that "at first, writing up the tasks with the group members was difficult and entailed a lot of effort". Ron also addressed this issue:

> Most of my life, in school, at work, and at other times as well, I wasn't asked to create something out of nothing. Most of the time we are asked to follow the beaten path, according to the accepted norms. But this course made me understand the meaning of independent learning. Even though it was sometimes difficult, it was the only way I was able to think about this important manner.

Facilitation of Information Use

The challenge of relying on resources and conducting accurate research helped the students acquire important skills, as reflected in this category. For example, the students described how they used existing material and applied it to unfamiliar or future situations. Learning how to draw conclusions and apply them in a different field while considering the limitations of the research allowed the students to use established sources when proposing solutions to their new problem. For example, Miriam stated:

> While seeking a solution to the problem, I began to understand that we don't have to develop what's already been established when dealing with current or future problems. Rather, we need to look around and realize what "there is" and what already exists, either in technological developments or in older products, to check how to make adjustments, changes or combinations according to the demands of the problem solutions.

The Development of Critical Literacy Skills

The students became aware that they needed to apply critical judgment in evaluating the information they found, to filter through it, and to choose only information that was appropriate. For example, Shon said:

> The difficulty I encountered in the area of innovation entailed filtering the information and not finding it. The notion of "a positronic brain" that serves as the central processing unit of an android has been in the literature since the 1940s, although as science fiction. Over the years, countless stories, novels, articles, and movies have been written in the field of robotics. When we investigated the topic, I discovered quite a lot of material that was new to me, but we had to learn what we could use.

Similarly, Luna wrote:

> The question that arose was whether this solution was relevant only for COVID-19 or whether we could use this solution in other situations that entail similar problems. After we researched and thoroughly read all the components of the solution, we decided to use it.

The students claimed that the learning method in this program offered them the advantages of active learning while also promoting their creativity and literacy skills, which they could use in the future in various fields, beyond the specific topics of the course. Moon wrote:

> I think the advantages of this learning approach for students are that it gives them new tools that in the past they would not have acquired at university. Until now, most of the courses I took felt like a kind of input–output; that is, you come to class and absorb material that has been circulating for years, up to the final exam, when you review a pool of questions from previous years, and during the exam you spit out everything you have accumulated. This not only fails to teach you effectively but also limits your creativity in particular and your way of thinking in general. All this undermines a thinking pattern geared to giving solutions to problems that may emerge in the future.

Contribution of the Task Sequence

The intervention program forced the students to work through a series of tasks, each of which emerged from the previous task. Continuous creativity demands focused thinking and methodological research. The series of tasks encouraged the learners to acquire and apply tools and provided them immediate feedback. The students reported that this process served as a smooth path to finding solutions and inspired actions that involved critical literacy and information filtering. Limor commented on this topic:

> The fact that the tasks were based on each other, that is, were in a sequence, maintained continuity of thought and therefore helped me when submitting the assignments. I felt the sequence of the assignments constructed my thinking.

Ari similarly wrote:

> As I noted, one of the most prominent advantages was the fact that all tasks so far have been based on each other. For example, in the first task, we were asked to raise problems we think may arise in the future during the era of telemedicine. In task 2 we already had to search for solutions to our problems. Picking a certain topic and focusing more and more on its details maintains the continuity of your train of though. [This keeps me] focused so I don't get lost in the assignments and supplementary material.

Using computer technologies to complete their tasks proved advantageous for the students. These technologies tapped into their development of functional literacy skills, such as seeking and finding materials, as well as of interactive literacy skills that make use of digital information and competencies. The students reported that using these tools enhanced their digital abilities and enriched their knowledge about digital tools. Mariya wrote:

> Thanks to the poster assignment, I learned how to use two new computer programs, ThingLink and Piktochart, and I really enjoyed learning about and using them. I learned how to write the information and material in a focused and practical manner and present all the relevant information we want to present.

Ari commented:

> We found Piktochart to be inconvenient in Hebrew, and I didn't feel comfortable with the visual design of the poster we created. Therefore, after another meeting, we decided to change the design and work with a different software. I suggested to my teammates that we incorporate the possibilities offered by the ThingLink software into the poster, and we used this software to build the poster until we were satisfied with the design. We wanted our poster presentation to be innovative, interesting and include all the material.

The challenges of the project and the work in diverse groups enabled the students to examine and experience these processes from the perspective of other student populations. Looking at things from alternative perspectives is an important part of handling different levels of literacy among the general population and students. For example, Ron noted:

Creating a heterogenous group made up of people from different social, educational, gender and other backgrounds will generate diverse thinking and different perspectives on the challenge, diminishing the option of cognitive stability… not to fixate on a certain area and search only there, [but] to examine cooperation and unconventional thinking directions and to look at the material from varying perspectives.

This study examined the experiences and perceptions of students who were trained in online digital literacy using FBL methodology. The three levels of literacy—functional, interactive, and evaluative—were manifested in their reflective journals. The students stated that the learning methods improved their skills in looking up information, understanding relevant medical material, taking action, and interacting with their peers to create a final online health-related project using digital tools. Furthermore, their evaluative literacy skills developed as they practiced assessing and filtering the available information and engaged in peer judgment.

Discussion

The important role of digitalization in healthcare has become apparent in the past decade, particularly during the COVID-19 pandemic and its aftermath (Alt & Naamati-Schneider, 2021). In light of this reality, those in charge of education in healthcare management and other medical fields must make the development of medical literacy among students a priority.

This chapter proposed using FPS together with effective instruction as a constructive pedagogic tool and demonstrated how this method can be used online to promote eHealth literacy among students at the outset of their academic training. Previous research on students' problem-solving and digital literacy skills found that students tend to possess only limited and basic digital literacy skills and limited knowledge about how to use information and communication technologies (Frank & Castek, 2017; Ozdamar-Keskin et al., 2015; Quann, 2015; Vanek, 2017). The study described in this chapter proposes a way to promote digital skills among students using the well-structured six sequential steps of the FPS pedagogical method.

The analysis of the students' reflective diaries revealed four main categories: (1) ability to search for and find material; (2) facilitation of information use; (3) development of critical literacy skills; and (4) contribution of task sequence. The findings underscore the importance of using this method during online or hybrid learning to promote and develop eHealth literacy on the functional, interactive, and evaluative levels. They also highlight the value of instructor guidance for students in the health professions as they learn to develop eHealth literacy abilities.

The six sequential steps of the FPS pedagogical method together with effective instruction enabled the students to locate material relevant to their studies, consider information critically, filter it, and choose only what is appropriate. The series of tasks encouraged them to acquire and use tools and receive immediate feedback. The use of computer technologies improved their digital skills and enriched their knowledge of digital tools, thus enhancing their functional literacy. By working in diverse groups, they were able to gain alternative perspectives, practice evaluation and filtering of available information, and carry out peer assessment.

Indeed, the findings of this study highlight the changing role of academia in medical education. In today's reality, academic institutions must produce graduates who are well-prepared to adapt to the changing environment of the medical world and the demands of the healthcare system and general workforce in the twenty-first century.

Academic institutions must devise constructivist learning methods and strategies to develop these needs in online settings. Moreover, they must recognize the role of instructors as learning facilitators who strive to design successful scaffolding strategies to promote students' health knowledge and cultivate their digital literacy, as part of lifelong learning skills essential in today's world.

References

Alt, D., & Raichel, N. (2020). Enhancing perceived digital literacy skills and creative self-concept through gamified learning environments: Insights from a longitudinal study. *International Journal of Educational Research, 101*, 101561.https://doi.org/10.1016/j.ijer.2020.101561

Alt, D., Naamati-Schneider, L., & Meirovich, A. (2022). Future problem-solving practiced during COVID-19: Implications for health management students' E-health literacy identity. *Frontiers in Psychology*, 13. https://doi.org/10.3389/fpsyg.2022.829243

Alt, D., & Naamati-Schneider, L. (2021). Health management students' self-regulation and digital concept mapping in online learning environments. *BMC Medical Education, 21*, 110. https://doi.org/10.1186/s12909-021-02542-w

Alt, D., & Naamati-Schneider, L. (2022). Online argumentation-based learning aided by digital concept mapping during COVID-19: Implications for health management teaching and learning. *Health Education, 122*, 18–36. https://doi.org/10.1108/HE-12-2020-0125

Berkhout, J. J., Helmich, E., Teunissen, P. W., van der Vleuten, C. P., & Jaarsma, A. D. C. (2018). Context matters when striving to promote active and lifelong learning in medical education. *Medical Education, 52*(1), 34–44. https://doi.org/10.1111/medu.13463

Cramond, B. L. (2009). Future problem solving in gifted education. In L. Shavinina (Ed.), *International handbook on giftedness* (pp. 1143–1156). Springer.

Deshpande, N., Arora, V. M., Vollbrecht, H., Meltzer, D. O., & Press, V. (2023). EHealth literacy and patient portal use and attitudes: Cross-sectional observational study. *JMIR Human Factors, 10*, e40105. https://doi.org/10.2196/40105

Diviani, N., van den Putte, B., Giani, S., & van Weert, J. C. (2015). Low health literacy and evaluation of online health information: A systematic review of the literature. *Journal of Medical Internet Research, 17*(5), e112. https://doi.org/10.2196/jmir.4018

El-Benny, M., Kabakian-Khasholian, T., El-Jardali, F., & Bardus, M. (2021). Application of the eHealth literacy model in digital health interventions: Scoping review. *Journal of Medical Internet Research, 23*(6), e23473. https://doi.org/10.2196/23473

Frank, T. H. J., & Castek, J. (2017). From digital literacies to digital problem solving: Expanding technology-rich learning opportunities for adults: The resource for adult education. *Journal of Research and Practice for Adult Literacy, Secondary, and Basic Education, 6*(2), 66–70.

Garcia, R., Falkner, K., & Vivian, R. (2018). Systematic literature review: Self-regulated learning strategies using e-learning tools for computer science. *Computers & Education, 123*, 150–163. https://doi.org/10.1016/j.compedu.2018.05.006

Guba, E., & Lincoln, Y. (2002). Paradigmas en competencia en la investigación cualitativa. *Por los rincones. Antología de métodos cualitativos en la investigación social*, 113–145.

Hemmo-Lotem, M., Tzezana, R., & Levtzion-Korach, O. (2021). The information revolution in medicine. *Hrefuaa (The Medicine), 160*, 24–29. (Hebrew).

Hemmo-Lotem, M., & Shani, M. (2018). Changing the paradigm in medicine in the wake of the fourth industrial revolution. *Hrefuaa (The Medicine), 157*, 797–801. (Hebrew).

Jarva, E., Oikarinen, A., Andersson, J., Tomietto, M., Kääriäinen, M., & Mikkonen, K. (2023). Healthcare professionals' digital health competence and its core factors; development and psychometric testing of two instruments. *International Journal of Medical Informatics*, 104995. https://doi.org/10.1016/j.ijmedinf.2023.104995

Kaper, M. S., Reijneveld, S. A., van Es, F. D., de Zeeuw, J., Almansa, J., Koot, J., & de Winter, A. F. (2019). Effectiveness of a comprehensive health literacy consultation skills training for undergraduate medical students: A randomized controlled trial. *International Journal of Environmental Research and Public Health, 17*(1), 81. https://doi.org/10.3390/ijerph17010081

Kebritchi, M., Lipschuetz, A., & Santiague, L. (2017). Issues and challenges for teaching successful online courses in higher education: A literature review. *Journal of Educational Technology Systems, 46*(1), 4–29. https://doi.org/10.1177/0047239516661713

Khan, N., Sarwar, A., Chen, T. B., & Khan, S. (2022). Connecting digital literacy in higher education to the 21st century workforce. *Knowledge Management & E-Learning,* 14(1), 46–61. https://doi.org/10.34105/j.kmel.2022.14.004

Kim, R., Olfman, L., Ryan, T., & Eryilmaz, E. (2014). Leveraging a personalized system to improve self-directed learning in online educational environments. *Computers & Education, 70*, 150–160. https://doi.org/10.1016/j.compedu.2013.08.006

Kraus, S., Schiavone, F., Pluzhnikova, A., & Invernizzi, A. C. (2021). Digital transformation in healthcare: Analyzing the current state-of-research. *Journal of Business Research, 123*, 557–567. https://doi.org/10.1016/j.jbusres.2020.10.030

Lopez, L., & Grant, R. W. (2012). Closing the gap: Eliminating health care disparities among Latinos with diabetes using health information technology tools and patient navigators. *Journal of Diabetes Science and Technology., 6*, 169–176. https://doi.org/10.1177/193229681200600121

Maeda, K., & Socha-Dietrich, K. (2021). Skills for the future health workforce: Preparing health professionals for people-centred care. *OECD Health Working Papers, No. 124*. https://doi.org/10.1787/68fb5f08-en

Main, L. F., Delcourt, M. A., & Treffinger, D. J. (2019). Effects of group training in problem-solving style on future problem-solving performance. *The Journal of Creative Behavior, 53*(3), 274–285. https://doi.org/10.1002/jocb.176

Marques, I. C. P., & Ferreira, J. J. M. (2020). Digital transformation in the area of health: Systematic review of 45 years of evolution. *Health and Technology, 10*(3), 575–586. https://doi.org/10.1007/s12553-019-00402-8

Mehoudar, O. (2014). Health literacy, and eHealth literacy: Access to health information as a key to equal opportunity in society. *Kidum Briut in Israel (The Advancement of Health in Israel), 5*, 25–34. (Hebrew).

Mitsutake, S., Shibata, A., Ishii, K., & Oka, K. (2016). Associations of eHealth literacy with health behavior among adult internet users. *Journal of Medical Internet Research, 18*(7), e192. https://doi.org/10.2196/jmir.5413

Mullan, J., Burns, P., Weston, K., McLennan, P., Rich, W., Crowther, S., Mansfield, K., et al. (2017). Health literacy amongst health professional university students: A study using the health literacy questionnaire. *Education Sciences, 7*(2), 54. https://doi.org/10.3390/educsci7020054

Naamati Schneider, L. (2020). Strategic management as adaptation to changes in the ecosystems of public hospitals in Israel. *Israel Journal of Health Policy Research, 9*(1), 1–11. https://doi.org/10.1186/s13584-020-00424-y

Naamati-Schneider, L. (2022). Intraorganisation conflicts of interest in hospitals adapting to a changing ecosystem. *Journal of Health Organisation and Management, 36*(3), 265–278. https://doi.org/10.1108/jhom-09-2021-0325

Naamati-Schneider, L., & Salvatore, F. P. (2022). Digital transformation in private dental clinics. In *Business advancement through technology volume I: Markets and marketing in transition* (pp. 201–218). Springer International Publishing. https://doi.org/10.1007/978-3-031-07769-2_10

Naamati-Schneider, L., & Salvatore, F. P. (2023). Sustainability for healthcare organisations and systems: Cultivating strategy and governance processes for a better future. In D. Vrontis, A. Thrassou, L. Efthymiou, Y. Weber, S. M. R. Shams, & E. Tsoukatos (Eds.), *Business for sustainability, volume I. Palgrave studies in cross-disciplinary business research.* In Association with EuroMed Academy of Business. Palgrave Macmillan. https://doi.org/10.1007/978-3-031-37361-9_11

Naamati-Schneider, L., & Zaks, O. (2022). Public hospitals in crisis: Managerial and strategic adaptation. In D. Vrontis, A. Thrassou, Y. Weber, S. M. R. Shams, E. Tsoukatos, & L. Efthymiou (Eds.), *Business under crisis, volume II. Palgrave studies in cross-disciplinary business research.* In Association with EuroMed Academy of Business. Palgrave Macmillan. https://doi.org/10.1007/978-3-030-76575-0_3

Naamati-Schneider, L. (2023). The effect of digitalization on service orientation and service perception among Israeli healthcare professionals: A qualitative study. *Digital Health, 9*. https://doi.org/10.1177/20552076231191892

Nagler, R. H., Ramanadhan, S., Minsky, S., & Viswanath, K. (2013). Recruitment and retention for community-based eHealth interventions with populations of low socioeconomic position: Strategies and challenges. *The Journal of Communication, 63*, 201–220. https://doi.org/10.1111/jcom.12008

National Institute for Literacy. (1991). *National Literacy Act*. Retrieved from https://www.congress.gov/bill/102nd-congress/house-bill/

Nguyen, H. T., Do, B. N., Pham, K. M., Kim, G. B., Dam, H., Nguyen, T. T., Nguyen, T., Nguyen, Y. H., Sørensen, K., Pleasant, A., & Duong, T. V. (2020). Fear of COVID-19 scale-associations of its scores with health literacy and health-related behaviors among medical students. *International Journal of Environmental Research and Public Health, 17*(11), 4164. https://doi.org/10.3390/ijerph17114164

Norman, C. D., & Skinner, H. A. (2006). EHealth literacy: Essential skills for consumer health in a networked world. *Journal of Medical Internet Research, 8*(2), e9.

Nutbeam, D., & McGill, B. (2019). Improving health literacy in clinical and community populations. In *International Handbook of Health Literacy: Research, practice and policy across the lifespan.* Policy Press.

Ozdamar-Keskin, N., Ozata, F. Z., Banar, K., & Royle, K. (2015). Examining digital literacy competences and learning habits of open and distance learners. *Contemporary Educational Technology, 6*(1), 74–90. https://doi.org/10.30935/cedtech/6140

Paakkari, L., & Okan, O. (2020). COVID-19: Health literacy is an underestimated problem. *The Lancet. Public Health, 5*(5), e249–e250. https://doi.org/10.1016/S2468-2667(20)30086-4

Quann, S. (2015). *Integrating digital literacy and problem solving into instruction.* LINCS Regional Professional Development Center for Adult Education. Retrieved from http://www.worlded.org

Rueda-Medina, B., Gómez-Urquiza, J. L., Casas-Barragán, A., Toledano-Moreno, S., Aguilar-Ferrándiz, M. E., & Correa-Rodríguez, M. (2023). eHealth literacy, internet use and health-related behaviour among health sciences students: A cross sectional study: eHealth literacy, internet use and health-related behaviour. *Contemporary Nurse*, 1–16. https://doi.org/10.1080/10376178.2023.2166547

Schwab, K. (2017). *The fourth industrial revolution.* Currency.

Sørensen, K., Pelikan, J. M., Röthlin, F., Ganahl, K., Slonska, Z., Doyle, G., Fullam, J., Kondilis, B., Agrafiotis, D., Uiters, E., Falcon, M., Mensing, M., Tchamov, K., van den Broucke, S., & Brand, H. (2015). Health literacy in Europe: Comparative results of the European health literacy survey (HLS-EU). *European Journal of Public Health, 25*(6), 1053–1058. https://doi.org/10.1093/eurpub/ckv043

Stellefson, M., Hanik, B., Chaney, B., Chaney, D., Tennant, B., & Chavarria, E. A. (2011). EHealth literacy among college students: A systematic review with implications for eHealth education. *Journal of Medical Internet Research, 13*, e102. https://doi.org/10.2196/jmir.1703

Tennant, B., Stellefson, M., Dodd, V., Chaney, B., Chaney, D., Paige, S., & Alber, J. (2015). eHealth literacy and Web 2.0 health information seeking behaviors among baby boomers and older adults. *Journal of Medical Internet Research, 17*(3), e70. https://doi.org/10.2196/jmir.3992

Topol, E. (2012). *The creative destruction of medicine: How the digital revolution will create better health care*. Basic Books.

Torrance, E. P., & Cramond, B. (2002). Needs of creativity programs, training, and research in the schools of the future. *Research in the Schools, 9*(2), 5–14.

Treffinger, D. J., Schoonover, P. F., & Selby, E. C. (2021). *Educating for creativity and innovation: A comprehensive guide for research-based practice*. Routledge.

Tripto, J., Ben-Zvi Assaraf, O., Snapir, Z., & Amit, M. (2016). The 'What is a system' reflection interview as a knowledge integration activity for high school students' understanding of complex systems in human biology. *International Journal of Science Education, 38*, 564–595.

UNESCO. (2018). Digital skills critical for job and social inclusion. Retrieved from https://en.unesco.org/news/digital-skills-critical-jobs-and-social-inclusion

Vanek, J. (2017). Using the PIAAC framework for problem solving in technology-rich environments to guide instruction: An introduction for adult educators. Retrieved from https://static1.squarespace.com

Veikkolainen, P., Tuovinen, T., Jarva, E., Tuomikoski, A. M., Männistö, M., Pääkkönen, J., Pihlajasalo T., & Reponen, J. (2023). eHealth competence building for future doctors and nurses–Attitudes and capabilities. *International Journal of Medical Informatics, 169*, 104912. https://doi.org/10.1016/j.ijmedinf.2022.104912

Walters, R., Leslie, S. J., Polson, R., et al. (2020). Establishing the efficacy of interventions to improve health literacy and health behaviours: A systematic review. *BMC Public Health, 20*, 1040. https://doi.org/10.1186/s12889-020-08991-0

WHO. (2019, June 2022). World Health Organisation: Universal health coverage. Retrieved from https://www.who.int/news-room/fact-sheets/detail/universal-health-coverage-(uhc)

Xie, B. (2011). Effects of an eHealth literacy intervention for older adults. *Journal of Medical Internet Research, 13*, e90. https://doi.org/10.2196/jmir.1880

Yang, S. C., Luo, Y. F., & Chiang, C. H. (2017). The associations among individual factors, eHealth literacy, and health-promoting lifestyles among college students. *Journal of Medical Internet Research, 19*(1), e15. https://doi.org/10.2196/jmir.5964

Yin, R. K. (2012). Case study methods. In H. Cooper, P. M. Camic, D. L. Long, A. T. Panter, D. Rindskopf, & K. J. Sher (Eds.), *APA handbook of research methods in psychology, vol. 2. Research designs: Quantitative, qualitative, neuropsychological, and biological* (pp. 141–155). American Psychological Association. https://doi.org/10.1037/13620-009

Zohar, A., & Barzilai, S. (2013). A review of research on metacognition in science education: Current and future directions. *Studies in Science Education, 49*, 121–169.

Part III
Intrapersonal Competencies

Chapter 7
Healthcare Management Students' Self-regulation Skills: Helping Students Become Proactive Learners

Abstract Adapting to the evolving healthcare market requires healthcare professionals to cultivate self-regulated learning (SRL) skills. This chapter examines the integration of SRL into the medical curriculum, emphasizing its importance in promoting proactive learning, enhancing metacognitive skills, and increasing motivation. It highlights the use of reflective journal writing as an educational tool to foster SRL and deepen engagement with learning materials. This approach aids in developing personal identity and influencing practice, ultimately preparing students for professional challenges and fostering a skilled, adaptable, and resilient workforce.

Introduction

The twenty-first century is characterized by the rapid accumulation of knowledge as well as by numerous and profound changes, developments, and advances in complex technologies that are exerting control over many spheres of our lives. These widespread changes have also had an impact upon the medical profession. Indeed, the healthcare system and its professionals are constantly called upon to cope with dynamic changes and new challenges that require adapting the system to the ever-changing reality. These challenges are linked to the growing use of advanced technology and artificial intelligence and to the changing nature and scope of the medical and nursing professions (Jungwirth & Haluza, 2019; Naamati-Schneider, 2023). At the same time, the healthcare system must also adapt to the introduction of many new regulations and reforms, the lengthening of the human lifespan, and various demographic changes. Moreover, the medical field must respond to market conditions characterized by diminishing and limited resources and growing competition among multiple entities, including doctors themselves (Naamati-Schneider & Salvatore, 2023; van Houten-Schat et al., 2018). Accordingly, healthcare management and staff need a new set of qualifications that include flexibility, adaptability, planning ability, and self-regulation of learning (SRL). Indeed, in the twenty-first century these capabilities are becoming essential for doctors to do their jobs (Berkhout et al., 2018).

L. Naamati-Schneider and D. Alt, *Technology and Competency-Oriented Learning*,
https://doi.org/10.1007/978-981-97-5771-8_7

Accordingly, modern-day medical education has begun to focus on cultivating these lifelong learning skills in order to train medical managers and doctors to adapt to the new era and its demands. Among these skills, SRL has been deemed essential for doctors and healthcare professionals. SRL enables healthcare professionals to be flexible and to adjust to the dynamic changes characterizing the health market worldwide (Bransen et al., 2020). Hence, healthcare education programs must begin to develop tools and methods that can support healthcare students in developing their SRL, thereby helping them engage in proactive learning on the behavioral, metacognitive and motivational levels. In view of the importance of developing and assimilating these abilities among professionals and students in the medical field, the present chapter focuses on promoting SRL through reflective journal writing. Encouraging students to engage in reflective practices has been acknowledged as an essential goal in higher education that can enhance students' SRL and effectively prepare them for their subsequent professional experiences (Alt & Raichel, 2021; Alt et al., 2022; Nückles et al., 2020).

Self-regulation of Learning in Healthcare Curricula

For healthcare professionals, SRL is considered a core competence that is essential for safeguarding patient care (Lajoie et al., 2019). Practitioners and trainees in the health professions are expected to engage in self-regulation of their learning and practice. For example, in the context of today's rapidly and constantly changing medical world, medical professionals must ensure high standards in patient care provision. Doctors are responsible for determining their own learning needs and pursuing professional development opportunities, and medical residents are expected to identify their knowledge gaps and seek help from supervisors when needed (Bransen et al., 2020). To this end, they must continuously develop their competencies, define their own learning needs, set personal goals, and engage in appropriate learning activities. In effect, they must become self-regulated learners (Lucieer et al., 2016).

For students, SRL refers to the ability to understand their own learning (Schunk & Zimmerman, 1994) and to exert metacognitive, motivational, and behavioral control over their own learning processes (Zimmerman & Moylan, 2009). Metacognitive control is defined as the regulation of skills for planning, monitoring, and modifying awareness and control of one's thought processes (i.e., cognition). Self-regulated learners use cognitive strategies designed to enhance the encoding, understanding, and/or retention of learning and to pursue academic goals and regulatory strategies that enable them to self-monitor and control their own learning (Zimmerman & Martinez-Pons, 1986). Motivational control entails regulation of beliefs and attitudes, self-efficacy, perceived task difficulty, task value beliefs, and personal interest in the task (Pintrich & Schunk, 2002). Behavioral control refers to learners' ability to react to and regulate their behavior in the context of further learning processes.

Despite the importance of SRL for students, very little theoretical research has examined how undergraduate and/or postgraduate medical students regulate their learning (van Houten-Schat et al., 2018). Alt and Naamati-Schneider (2021), for example, showed how learners who were highly self-regulated were accustomed to setting standards for their assignments in online courses. They set short-term as well as long-term goals, maintained a high standard for their learning and the quality of their work in online courses, and undertook extra problems to master the content. These students were also more receptive to adopting innovative learning methods and tools, such as concept mapping to solve contemporary problems during online courses, and demonstrated a tendency to utilize such learning strategies. Indeed, they already assessed their own performance to varying degrees, while actively generating self-feedback and consciously controlling their own cognitive, affective, motivational, and behavioral learning. Alt and Naamati-Schneider (2021) further showed how SRL developed among the students by the end of the problem-based online activity. These researchers claimed that active learning enables students in the medical and health management professions to develop and acquire self-directed learning abilities. Acquiring these abilities constitutes an additional step toward adapting the health system and its practitioners to the demands and needs of the twenty-first century. Hence, the researchers concluded that although the effects of innovative interventions may vary depending upon learners' abilities, such learning strategies can further enhance students' SRL.

Teachers need to recognize and account for different types of learners and developmental levels of students, adapting their curricula and learning environment accordingly. This adaptation will encourage and scaffold students' effective use of self-regulated learning (SRL) strategies. For example, teachers can help struggling students create study schedules, thereby guiding their learning process toward goals that emphasize successful acquisition of skills and knowledge. Learners with low self-regulation may fail to see the advantages of innovative learning tools and methods. Providing such students with well-defined assessment criteria in advance may motivate them to invest adequate time and effort in the required tasks. Students with inadequate SRL skills may need to be further apprised of the benefits of such activities.

Other research studies indicated that students often have difficulty regulating their learning in clinical learning environments due to the unpredictable, dynamic and disorganized nature of clinical workplace settings (Bransen et al., 2020). Hence, healthcare curricula must support self-regulation as a central learning outcome by designing constructivist-based learning environments, thus helping students become more proactive by exerting metacognitive, motivational, and behavioral control over their own learning processes.

Supporting Self-regulation of Learning by Reflective Journal Writing

The above review prompts the following fundamental question: How can students' SRL be nurtured? In an attempt to answer this question in the context of the healthcare professions, prior studies have pointed to specific assessment practices aimed at promoting this important skill. One such practice is reflective journal (RJ) writing, a practice that has been deemed important for students in today's fluid and changing environment. Students must learn to manage their capabilities in a meaningful manner and reorient themselves to gain a sense of agency (Ryan, 2015). Making effective choices requires adopting a reflective approach to learning. Hence, lifelong learning generally necessitates self-regulation as well as self-assessment, which entails utilizing information and feedback from multiple sources. Schön (1983) maintained that through reflection, practitioners can make sense of uncertain situations.

Reflective journals are defined as "written documents that students create as they think about various concepts, events, or interactions over a period of time for the purposes of gaining insights into self-awareness and learning" (Thorpe, 2004, p. 328). Journal writing is related to metacognition as it "slows the pace of learning, increases the sense of ownership of learning, and ... has been described as a bridge across which learners can move from the specific to the general, while developing a habit of reflection" (Cowan, 2014. p. 54).

Indeed, journal writing is a tool that can be used to express self-observation of the learning process and to provide evidence of reflection (Wallin & Adawi, 2018). An essential benefit of this assessment tool is that it creates an environment in which students feel safe in expressing their concerns and exploring their thoughts. They are encouraged to reflect on the beliefs, values, experiences, and assumptions that influence their learning and to examine their development and progress over time (Minott, 2008). RJs can also affect behavior. According to Fabriz et al. (2014), during the reflection stage learners evaluate their work and judge whether their goal has been attained. Based on their assessment, they react and regulate their behavior in the context of further learning processes. Thus, the outcome of prior learning informs subsequent learning.

Metacognitive reflection dimensions are considered to be core competencies for healthcare professionals (Lajoie et al., 2019). Medical residents are expected to identify their own knowledge gaps and to seek help from supervisors when they need it (Bransen et al., 2020). To this end, they must continuously define their own learning needs, set personal goals, and engage in learning activities that are the most precise and appropriate for them. In essence, they must self-regulate their learning and become active participants in their own learning processes (Lucieer et al., 2016). Therefore, self-regulated learning (SRL) is considered a core competence that is essential for safeguarding patient care (Alt & Naamati-Schneider, 2021).

Despite the importance of these reflection components, students often have trouble regulating their learning in clinical learning environments (Bransen et al., 2020;

Lucieer et al., 2016). As students begin their clinical training, they often struggle with patient and medical staff interactions and need to apply their learned knowledge in the workplace using self-directed learning approaches. Moreover, during their early years in medicine, medical personnel face increased responsibilities and the need for independent task management. Effective patient care and self-directed learning skills are crucial during this period (Teunissen & Westerman, 2011). To support these needs, healthcare curricula are increasingly emphasizing metacognitive reflection through teaching reflective writing, helping students make sense of their experiences (Rajhans et al., 2020).The use of RJs to encourage higher-order thinking skills is now being investigated in higher education research and practice (Alt & Raichel, 2021). Engaging students in reflective practices has been recognized as a central learning goal that can effectively prepare students for their future professional lives, improve their lifelong learning and professional practice, help them function effectively in a diverse and complex practice environment and enable them to gain pedagogical insights from learning activities.

Research highlights the necessity for prompts to enhance student reflection on their learning processes in reflective journals (RJs). Molee et al. (2011) evaluated the depth of learning and critical thinking in service-learning courses at a public university, using prompting questions to assist students in assessing their academic enhancement, personal growth, and civic engagement. Students responded to specific prompts that facilitated objective descriptions and analytical evaluations of their experiences. The study also employed questions to help students refine their reflections, such as setting goals to improve themselves and the quality of their learning and future experiences (p. 243). The researchers found that asking prompting questions was useful in documenting student learning. Nevertheless, students had trouble applying critical evaluation to their own learning and thinking. The authors attributed these limitations to the novelty of the tool and the participants' insufficient experience with reflection processes. Krauskopf et al. (2018) also found that prompting questions to be useful in stimulating reflective discussion, in engaging participants in metacognitive development, and in enabling them to generate subjective interpretations of their knowledge, thus supporting their individualized growth.

Reflective Writing Scheme

Drawing on metacognition theory, the Learning to Learn Project (2002), and the recent Assessment Tools for Higher Education Learning Environments (ASSET, 2020) ERASMUS + project teams, Alt and Raichel (2021) created a bank of prompt questions that were systematically organized around three dimensions of metacognitive abilities essential for independent reflective learners: awareness, evaluation, and regulation. Awareness, or metacognitive knowledge, describes a state in which people are aware of what they know (tasks, specific knowledge). Evaluation entails thinking about the effectiveness and limitations of one's mind and the effectiveness of one's chosen strategy. Metacognitive regulation describes a state in which individuals think about their strategic planning and goal setting and the actions that must be taken in order to learn.

The affective dimension of learning involves students' emotions and how they manage them during learning processes. Pekrun and Loderer (2020) explored this relationship using control-value theory, categorizing emotions into achievement, epistemic, topic, and social. Their review primarily draws on studies from technology-enhanced environments like intelligent tutoring systems and simulations. They also examined learning from multiple perspectives, such as contradictory viewpoints in texts, and concluded with suggestions for future research and practical applications. Beyond the cognitive and affective levels, learning must involve the learner's active engagement to produce ongoing benefits for both the learner and the work or learning environment. Because critical reflection is only achieved if action ensues, reflective learning processes should prompt deliberative action. Indeed, metacognitive thinking skills alone cannot address the social contexts and structures that influence learning. Thus, these processes should include a reflective interplay between individuals and social structures to understand and change individuals' chosen courses of action (Ryan, 2015).

Based on their research, Alt and Raichel (2021) proposed the following two-dimensional reflection scheme. The first dimension entails students' current experiences or "short-term reflections" and deals with students' in-process experiences during the course. This reflection encompassed the following levels:

1. Cognitive—relates to the content of the course, learning skills, and learning purposes.
2. Behavioral—refers to students' behavior during the learning process.
3. Affective (emotional)—pertains to emotions arising during the learning experience.

As noted, the dimension of short-term reflections entails exploring a specific and immediate learning experience. The second dimension, in contrast, focuses on students' reflections on their learning experiences over the long term from the perspective of:

1. Academic development.
2. Professional development.
3. Personal development.
4. Multicultural development.

In addition, the scheme also stressed three essential metacognitive abilities:

1. Awareness of one's learning experience.
2. Evaluation of the learning experience.
3. Attitude and behavior regulation to perform better in the future.

Based on this theoretical framework, Alt et al. (2022) devised the Reflective Journal Scale (RJs). The scale comprises 30 items divided into two sub-scales: short-term (16 items) and long-term (15 items), all scored on a Likert-type scale ranging from 1 = *not true at all* to 6 = *completely true.* Table 7.1 summarizes the theoretical scheme, including the questionnaire items designed to capture students' perceptions of the RJ writing process. Sample question: "Reflective journal writing helped me think of ways that can help me better understand the material or assignment".

Subsequent Adoption of Reflective Practices in Workplace

A central goal of education is to offer students learning experiences that are useful beyond the specific conditions of initial learning (Lobato, 2012). These experiences should be accompanied by reflective thinking that can instigate new ideas and actions for improvement. In this regard, Kolb (1984) proposed a model of experiential learning suggesting that learners must first reflect before they can move on to active experimentation. The model includes four cyclical stages of experiential learning: concrete experience, reflective observation, abstract conceptualization, and planning active experimentation. Kolb (1984) contends that "learners ... must be able to reflect on and observe their experiences from many perspectives (RO). They must be able to create concepts that integrate their observations into logically sound theories (AC), and they must be able to use these theories to make decisions and solve problems (AE)" (p. 30).

In effect, reflective practice encourages learners to continue to learn from experience, to bridge the gap between theory and practice and to become lifelong learners (Kolb, 1984). Based on this theory, Brown et al. (2011) claimed that reflection should be considered a prerequisite for transferring knowledge and skills across classroom and work contexts. He further suggested that incorporating tools for reflection when designing training programs can facilitate this transfer. Other researchers (Asfeldt et al., 2018; Morris, 2020; Slade et al., 2019) similarly underscored the importance of critical reflection in the process of learning and discussed its vital role as a mediator of meaning.

Griggs et al. (2018) examined the potential connection between reflective learning and the subsequent adoption of reflective practices at work. In their study they examined the RJs of 75 participants in a leadership development program and assessed their utility for facilitating and assessing transfer and evaluating training. Among other results, their findings suggested that organizational training can benefit from the use of reflective tools such as RJs both for evaluating training effectiveness and for enhancing transfer. The program participants were encouraged and taught to "see things differently" (p. 9), critically evaluate other perspectives and recognize the complexity of reality. Combining expert knowledge with instruction on how to use reflective tools led to the emergence of professionals who held more mature perspectives than those they held prior to the professional training program. Nevertheless, the researchers contended that the evidence supporting and informing reflective practice in curriculum interventions remains largely theoretical. They stressed the lack of empirical data showing that the development of reflection in an academic context has long-term and definitive benefits for most learners. Indeed, despite the vast literature

Table 7.1 Reflective writing scheme and the reflective journal scale (RJs) items

Dimension 1	Short-term reflections		
	Awareness	Evaluation	Regulation
Cognitive level	• Describe exactly what I was asked to do in the course (or educational assignment) • Describe the main issues raised during the course (or educational assignment)	• Evaluate what additional material I need to learn in order to successfully complete the course or assignment • Evaluate the purposes of the course or assignment (e.g., why do I need to learn the materials? what other purposes can be suggested) • Evaluate my understanding of the assignment or materials taught • Describe why it is important to study the material or to complete the educational assignment (specify learning goals)	• Think about my experiences during the course or assignment that improved my learning methods • Think of ways that can help me better understand the material or assignment
Behavioral level	• Describe how I learned (methods/ activities I used to learn the subject)	• Evaluate what worked well during the learning activity (e.g., during group work) • Evaluate problems that emerged during the learning activity (e.g., during group work)	• Think about whether the way I learned (for example, alone or in a group) is the best way to learn • Think about how to improve my learning methods
Emotions (affective level)	• Describe my feelings during the course or assignment (what did I like most/least)	• Evaluate the reason for the feelings that emerged during the course or assignment (why did I feel that way?)	• Think of ways to improve my feelings about the course or assignment (e.g., about the learning material, the ways of learning)

(continued)

Table 7.1 (continued)

Dimension 2	*Long-term reflections*		
	Awareness	Evaluation	Regulation
Academic development	• Describe what I as a learner found easy to implement during the course or assignment	• Evaluate what else can be done to better link the learning material to my prior knowledge	• Describe what material or issues in the course or assignment may be related to my prior knowledge (for example, things I learned in past courses) • Think of ways that can help me deal with difficulties (remove barriers) during learning activities
Professional development	• Describe how what I learned during the course (knowledge, skill) might help me (be useful) in my current or future work	• Evaluate how I can adapt what I learned during the course (knowledge, skill) to my current or future work (what should I add? what can I omit?)	• Think about the experiences I "gained" during the course that may be useful in my current or future work
Personal development	• Describe what I learned from the course or assignment on the personal level—about myself (e.g., what are my strengths, what should be improved?)	• Evaluate what I learned from my experience during the course or assignment about my potential (what can I achieve?) • Evaluate what I would like to improve in myself	• Think of ways I can use the insights about myself that emerged during the course or assignment to become a better person in the future
Multicultural development	• Describe the relationship between different cultures and the studied materials	• Evaluate what I learned from a cultural perspective	• Think about ways of linking the educational activity to students' culture (language, customs, history)

focusing on reflection in teaching and learning, there is very little empirical research evidence pointing to the actual impact of reflection.

Guiding students to reflect deeply on their learning can be seen as a further means of encouraging them to contextualize their learning in relation to their current academic and future professional lives (Adie & Tangen, 2015). Alt et al. (2022) corroborated this notion by showing how reflective writing may increase the transfer of knowledge and skills to future settings. Their study showed that health management students' favorable perceptions of the reflective writing skills they gained were positively connected to their tendency to transfer the skills to their professional and personal lives. Based on PLS models, the researchers showed how health managers underscored the importance of long-term reflective skills and expressed their intention to use these skills in their future professional lives. This finding implies that encouraging students to think about a learning experience in the context of their long-term development may increase their tendency to use reflective skills in their future careers. Consequently, having students reflect on their learning experiences and, more importantly, discover the potential links between these experiences and their intrapersonal and interpersonal development, may help them recognize the benefits of this tool and encourage them to apply RJ skills to future activities.

Discussion

Our current and previous work underscores the effectiveness of using a generic reflection scheme to identify the dimensions of reflective thinking and to measure students' perceptions of their reflective writing experiences. The connection between perceived reflective writing and students' tendency to transfer this skill to their future careers and personal lives should be recognized. Using a bank of prompting questions organized according to a validated theoretical scheme may help teachers choose questions to inspire and assess different levels of reflective thinking among their students, in accordance with learning outcomes set in advance. These questions can assist teachers structure the journals and help students properly understand and implement reflective thinking.

The studies discussed in this chapter may also serve to alleviate the main barrier in using reflective journal practices as formative assessment tools. Teachers see RJ as a time-consuming task that requires investing extra time in checking and providing feedback to large groups of students. Students require feedback to help them identify their strengths and weaknesses during the learning process. Moreover, feedback is beneficial for teachers in that it enables them to adapt their instructional strategies to learners with different abilities. To cope with the extra time required, teachers may introduce the proposed scheme slowly and administer the questions gradually. For instance, as part of an ongoing assignment, they can ask their students to submit several journal entries, each related to a different level or dimension in the scheme. Moreover, online learning environments can offer opportunities for reflection by helping students focus on learning and guiding their engagement in reflection. Reflection can be also combined with peer review (a form of reflective learning based on the theory of experiential learning—Kolb, 1984) and peer feedback to exert a positive influence on students' self-regulated learning outcomes (Yang, 2010).

Reflective writing has been identified as an effective pedagogical tool for stimulating flexibility, adaptability, planning ability, and self-regulation of learning among students. These capabilities are becoming an essential and inseparable part of the array of tasks required of professionals in the twenty-first century. The proposed validated generic scheme can be adapted and integrated into different curricula, thereby increasing the potential for infusing RJ instructional strategies into higher education curricula, improving the quality of reflection in student journals, and promoting lifelong learning skills.

Reflective journal writing is a valuable tool for helping students regulate their learning in clinical settings. At the outset of their clinical training, students often have difficulty interacting with patients and medical staff and must learn new material using self-directed methods. Additionally, medical staff must exhibit self-directed learning skills to provide safe and effective patient care. As a result, healthcare curricula should focus on supporting metacognitive reflection as a central learning outcome. Through reflective writing, students can confer meaning to their learning experiences, thus enabling them to transfer their knowledge to the workplace setting. This approach can aid in the development of the self-directed learning skills that are crucial for medical staff in the early years of their practice.

References

Adie, L., & Tangen, D. (2015). The use of multimodal technologies to enhance reflective writing in teacher education. In M. E. Ryan (Ed.), *Teaching reflective learning in higher education* (pp. 127–138). Springer.

Alt, D., & Raichel, N. (2021). *Equity and formative assessment in higher education: Advancing culturally responsive assessment*. Springer.

Alt, D., & Naamati-Schneider, L. (2021). Health management students' self-regulation and digital concept mapping in online learning environments. *BMC Medical Education*. https://doi.org/10.1186/s12909-021-02542-w

Alt, D., Raichel, N., & Naamati-Schneider, L. (2022). Higher education students' reflective journal writing and lifelong learning skills: Insights from an exploratory sequential study. *Frontiers in Psychology*. https://doi.org/10.3389/fpsyg.2021.707168

Asfeldt, M., Hvenegaard, G., & Purc-Stephenson, R. (2018). Group writing, reflection, and discovery: A model for enhancing learning on wilderness educational expeditions. *Journal of Experiential Education, 41*, 241–260. https://doi.org/10.1177/1053825917736330

Assessment Tools for Higher Education Learning Environments [ASSET]. (2020). *Erasmus+ capacity building in the field of higher education*. Erasmus+ programme of the European Union. https://www.asset-erasmus.com/

Berkhout, J. J., Helmich, E., Teunissen, P. W., van der Vleuten, C. P., & Jaarsma, A. D. C. (2018). Context matters when striving to promote active and lifelong learning in medical education. *Medical Education, 52*(1), 34–44. https://doi.org/10.1111/medu.13463

Bransen, D., Govaerts, M. J., Sluijsmans, D. M., & Driessen, E. W. (2020). Beyond the self: The role of co-regulation in medical students' self-regulated learning. *Medical Education, 54*(3), 234–241. https://doi.org/10.1111/medu.14018

Brown, T., McCracken, M., & O'Kane, P. (2011) 'Don't forget to write': How reflective learning journals can help to facilitate, assess and evaluate training transfer. *Human Resource Development International, 14*, 465–481. https://psycnet.apa.org/, https://doi.org/10.1080/13678868.2011.601595

Cowan, J. (2014). Noteworthy matters for attention in reflective journal writing. *Active Learning in Higher Education, 15*, 53–64. https://doi.org/10.1177/1469787413514647

Fabriz, S., Van Ewijk, C. D., Poarch, G., & Büttner, G. (2014). Fostering self-monitoring of university students by means of a standardized learning journal—A longitudinal study with process analyses. *European Journal of Psychology of Education, 29*(2), 239–255. https://doi.org/10.1007/s10212-013-0196-z

Griggs, V., Holden, R., Lawless, A., & Rae, J. (2018). From reflective learning to reflective practice: Assessing transfer. *Studies in Higher Education, 43*, 1172–1183. https://doi.org/10.1080/03075079.2016.1232382

Jungwirth, D., & Haluza, D. (2019). Information and communication technology and the future of healthcare: Results of a multi-scenario Delphi survey. *Health Informatics Journal, 25*(1), 161–173.

Kolb, D. A. (1984). *Experiential learning: Experience as the source of learning and development.* Prentice-Hall.

Krauskopf, K., Foulger, T. S., & Williams, M. K. (2018). Prompting teachers' reflection of their professional knowledge. A proof-of-concept study of the graphic assessment of TPACK instrument. *Teacher Development, 22*(2), 153–174. https://doi.org/10.1080/13664530.2017.1367717

Lajoie, S. P., Zheng, J., Li, S., Jarrell, A., & Gube, M. (2019). Examining the interplay of affect and self regulation in the context of clinical reasoning. *Learning and Instruction.* https://doi.org/10.1016/j.learninstruc.2019.101219

Learning to Learn Project. (2002). *Reflective learning journal (teacher guide).* The Hong Kong Polytechnic University. Retrieved from https://www.polyu.edu.hk/learn-to-learn/

Lobato, J. (2012). The actor-oriented transfer perspective and its contributions to educational research and practice. *Educational Psychologist, 47*, 232–247. https://psycnet.apa.org/, https://doi.org/10.1080/00461520.2012.693353

Lucieer, S. M., Jonker, L., Visscher, C., Rikers, R. M., & Themmen, A. P. (2016). Self-regulated learning and academic performance in medical education. *Medical Teacher, 38*(6), 585–593. https://doi.org/10.3109/0142159x.2015.1073240

Minott, M. A. (2008). Valli's typology of reflection and the analysis of pre-service teachers' reflective journals. *Australian Journal of Teacher Education, 33*(5), 55–65. https://doi.org/10.14221/ajte.2008v33n5.4

Molee, L. M., Henry, M. E., Sessa, V. I., & McKinney-Prupis, E. R. (2011). Assessing learning in service-learning courses through critical reflection. *Journal of Experiential Education, 33*(3), 239–257. https://doi.org/10.5193/JEE33.3.239

Morris, T. H. (2020). Experiential learning–a systematic review and revision of Kolb's model. *Interactive Learning Environments, 28*(8), 1064–1077. https://doi.org/10.1080/10494820.2019.1570279

Naamati-Schneider, L., & Salvatore, F. P. (2023). Sustainability for healthcare organisations and systems: Cultivating strategy and governance processes for a better future. In D. Vrontis, A. Thrassou, L. Efthymiou, Y. Weber, S. M. R. Shams, & E. Tsoukatos (Eds.), *Business for sustainability, volume I* (Palgrave Studies in Cross-disciplinary Business Research, In Association with EuroMed Academy of Business). Palgrave Macmillan. https://doi.org/10.1007/978-3-031-37361-9_11

Naamati-Schneider, L. (2023). The effect of digitalization on service orientation and service perception among Israeli healthcare professionals: A qualitative study. *Digital Health, 9*. https://doi.org/10.1177/20552076231191892

Nückles, M., Roelle, J., Glogger-Frey, I., Waldeyer, J., & Renkl, A. (2020). The self-regulation-view in writing-to-learn: Using journal writing to optimize cognitive load in self-regulated learning. *Educational Psychology Review, 32*(4), 1089–1126.

Pekrun, R., & Loderer, K. (2020). Emotions and learning from multiple representations and perspectives. In R. Pekrun & K. Loderer (Eds.), *Handbook of learning from multiple representations and perspectives* (pp. 373–400). Routledge.

Pintrich, P. R., & Schunk, D. H. (2002). *Motivation in education: Theory, research and applications.* Prentice Hall Merrill.

Rajhans, V., Eichler, R., Sztrigler-Cohen, O., & Gordon-Shaag, A. (2020). A novel method of enhancing students' involvement in reflective writing. *The Clinical Teacher*. https://doi.org/10.1111/tct.13303

Ryan, M. E. (Ed.). (2015). *Teaching reflective learning in higher education*. Springer.

Schön, D. A. (1983). *The reflective practitioner*. Basic Books.

Schunk, D. H., & Zimmerman, B. J. (Eds.). (1994). *Self-regulation of learning and performance: Issues and educational applications*. Lawrence Erlbaum Associates, Inc.

Slade, M. L., Burnham, T. J., Catalana, S. M., & Waters, T. (2019). The impact of reflective practice on teacher candidates' learning. *International Journal for the Scholarship of Teaching and Learning, 13*(2), 15. https://doi.org/10.20429/ijsotl.2019.130215

Teunissen, P. W., & Westerman, M. (2011). Opportunity or threat: The ambiguity of the consequences of transitions in medical education. *Medical Education, 45*(1), 51–59. https://doi.org/10.1111/j.1365-2923.2010.03755.x

Thorpe, K. (2004). Reflective learning journals: From concept to practice. *Reflective Practice, 5*, 328–343. https://doi.org/10.1080/1462394042000270655

Van Houten-Schat, M. A., Berkhout, J. J., van Dijk, N., Endedijk, M. D., Jaarsma, A. D. C., & Diemers, A. D. (2018). Self-regulated learning in the clinical context: A systematic review. *Medical Education, 52*(10), 1008–1015. https://doi.org/10.1111/medu.13615

Wallin, P., & Adawi, T. (2018). The reflective diary as a method for the formative assessment of self-regulated learning. *European Journal of Engineering Education, 43*, 507–521. https://doi.org/10.1080/03043797.2017.1290585

Yang, Y. F. (2010). Students' reflection on online self-correction and peer review to improve writing. *Computers & Education, 55*(3), 1202–1210. https://doi.org/10.1016/j.compedu.2010.05.017

Zimmerman, B. J., & Martinez-Pons, M. (1986). Development of a structured interview for assessing student use of self-regulated learning strategies. *American Educational Research Journal, 23*, 614–628. https://doi.org/10.3102/00028312023004614

Zimmerman, B. J., & Moylan, A. R. (2009). Self-regulation: Where metacognition and motivation intersect. In D. J. Hacker, J. Dunlosky, & A. C. Graesser (Eds.), *Handbook of metacognition in education* (pp. 299–315). Routledge.

Chapter 8
Ethical Judgment and Ethical Leadership in Healthcare Management Education

Abstract Navigating the ethical complexities of the healthcare market amid global ecosystem changes is increasingly vital. This chapter examines the impact of strategic and technological shifts on the ethical dimensions of healthcare. It underscores the need for ethical judgment, the creation of an ethical code for medical management, and the cultivation of ethical leadership. Various intervention programs promoting these competencies are described, covering all training levels from professional studies to in-service training within healthcare organizations. Developing ethical judgment among healthcare managers and organizations will foster trust, equity, and quality within the health system.

Introduction

The issue of ethics frequently appears on the public agenda, particularly in the field of healthcare. Indeed, healthcare professionals at all levels are confronted with ethical issues and dilemmas on a daily basis. Moreover, recent global and local changes have brought about diverse ethical and moral challenges that the healthcare system has been forced to deal with (see Chap. 2).

This chapter reviews changes in the healthcare market that have necessitated the application of ethical judgment, the construction of an ethical code for medical management, and the development of ethical leadership in the health field. Additionally, the chapter reviews issues of ethics, bioethics and medical ethics and examines relevant medical education and research in this field. It also discusses intervention programs for promoting and developing these competencies at all levels of training, from the outset of professional studies and via professional training offered within health organizations themselves. Inculcating and developing ethical judgment among healthcare professionals and managers can help generate trust in all parts of the system, including patients, thus strengthening the values of equity and quality in the health system.

L. Naamati-Schneider and D. Alt, *Technology and Competency-Oriented Learning*,
https://doi.org/10.1007/978-981-97-5771-8_8

Ethical Judgment, Moral Dilemmas, and the Need for Ethical Leadership Within an Ever-Changing Healthcare Environment

For many years healthcare professionals enjoyed a certain degree of autonomy. Yet this autonomy was limited by the formulation of an ethical code designed to regulate their conduct within the system and provide a moral framework for their actions, mainly for the benefit of patients. Across the globe, organizations of doctors and healthcare professionals have formulated various codes that supplement the Hippocratic Oath and constitute a framework for their actions. Such codes are constantly updated to accommodate changes in the environment (Hall et al., 2024; Karni & Reches, 2018; Khosravi et al., 2024; WMA Declaration of Geneva, 2017). Indeed, to respond to the mounting number of medical dilemmas in everyday practice, healthcare associations and organizations must engage in healthcare ethics such as the healthcare ethics consultation (HCEC) (Nagao & Takimoto, 2023). In Chap. 2 we described the macro-, meso- and micro-level changes in the environment of healthcare organizations that were described in that have compelled healthcare systems and medical management personnel to change their approach to administration and treatment. Here we contend that these changes must be assessed from an ethical as well as a legal standpoint (Ijiga et al., 2024; TerKonda & Fish, 2023; Karni & Reches, 2018). The following examples highlight some of the ethical decisions professionals in the healthcare field must address on a daily basis (McBride et al., 2018).

At the *macro* level, healthcare systems must consider issues such as allotting resources and setting priorities, determining public health policies, promoting health in the population, establishing regulations and standardization, balancing between private and public health systems, and confronting an assortment of ethical issues stemming from these perceptions and policies.

At the *meso* or organizational level, medical management personnel must make moral decisions and judgments on a daily basis concerning resource allotment, organizational manpower, management of medical professionals, professional responsibility, treatment provision and documentation, and ensuring medical continuity. Indeed, the strategic business processes they have had to adopt to maintain a marketing and service orientation are altering the character, vision, and objectives of health organizations, thus influencing their organizational culture.

Change frequently engenders an inherent conflict of interests and values within a system and its workers. Such contradicting values pose ethical and moral challenges that necessitate integration between financial and medical considerations, the provision of egalitarian medicine, and balancing between public and private medicine (Naamati-Schneider, 2021, 2022). Moreover, the digital transformation of healthcare systems has engendered new ethical issues and dilemmas. Among these are the digitalization and computerized handling of medical records and patient information, the provision of digital medicine, the question of medical responsibility in digital medicine, cyber threats, the need to ensure information security and preserve patient confidentiality, digital accessibility to treatment, retaining treatment continuity, documentation, and the use of long-distance communication (Karni & Reches, 2018; McBride et al, 2018; Naamati-Schneider, 2023; Naamati-Schneider et al., 2024a, 2024b; Olorunsogo et al., 2024). These changes will undoubtedly yield ethical advantages: Digital tools will reduce the gaps in treatment quality and wait times between peripheral and central regions, thus making healthcare services more equitable. Yet they also entail numerous disadvantages, such as adjustment and accessibility issues among weaker population groups and undermining the trust between doctors and patients. These complex moral difficulties and dilemmas must be handled at all levels.

At the *micro* or personal level, medical personnel must cope with an assortment of ethical issues emerging from modifications and new treatment methods, among them home hospitalization, long-distance treatment, technology use, and robotics. In addition, they must deal with contradictions between personal and organizational value perceptions and discrepancies between personal values of equality and treatment and organizational, financial, and profit considerations (Dean et al., 2019; Naamati-Schneider, 2022; Naamati-Schneider et al., 2024a, 2024b). The caregiver-patient relationship is also changing, as is the status of doctors, the extent of patient autonomy and patient involvement in treatment and decision-making, and the matter of medical confidentiality (Allen et al., 2024; Fenton et al., 2012; Präg et al., 2017). These changes have had immediate repercussions upon the extent of doctors' involvement and responsibility during treatment, requiring doctors to consider ethical issues when managing patients and cases (Powers & Bendall, 2004; Weizman, 2021, pp. 135–145). Numerous ethical dilemmas have emerged from the need to provide the best possible treatment while taking patient type and relationship type (paternalistic, informative, or cooperative) into consideration. For example, doctors' decision-making is liable to infringe upon patient autonomy. Doctors may also find themselves succumbing to financial pressures in deciding upon what treatment to offer when the main consideration should be what is most beneficial for the patient (McBride et al., 2015; Sulmasy et al., 2017).

The evolution of healthcare professionals' approach from paternalistic to more patient-centered care has raised various ethical concerns. These include the ethical implications of environmental factors affecting patients and influencing clinical decisions, as well as the adverse effects of caregiver boundaries, where healthcare providers may exert authority over patients, potentially compromising their autonomy. (Rathert et al., 2016; Weizman, 2021). The introduction of technological and digital treatment means can also disrupt the patient-caregiver relationship, engendering numerous ethical and moral dilemmas (Allen et al., 2024; Naamati-Schneider et al., 2024; Rathert et al., 2016). Such dilemmas require systems and the individuals within them to adapt their behavior and become more inclusive. Figure 8.1 summarizes the key ethical dilemmas outlined above, as manifested across all three levels of the healthcare system.

Figure 8.1 highlights the ethical challenges and complexities inherent in healthcare decision-making today and underscores the need for a systematic and multifaceted approach to these dilemmas. In light of these changes, we emphasize the importance of developing ethical leadership as well as of establishing an ethical

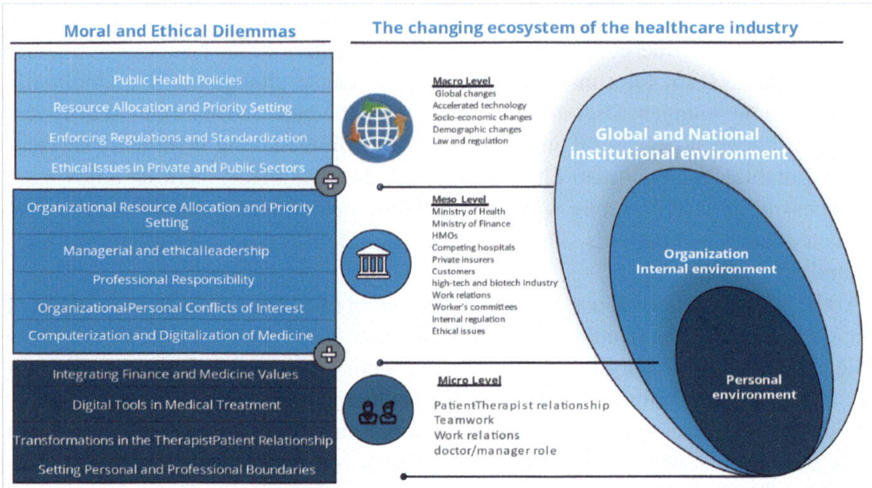

Fig. 8.1 Dilemmas across three levels of the healthcare system

framework for organizations in general and healthcare organizations in particular. Furthermore, a broad holistic vision is needed that takes into account all managerial and treatment considerations within health organizations and systems. The need for such a vision once again underscores the importance of offering programs to train healthcare professionals in ethical leadership and develop their awareness of this issue, while placing emphasis on decision-making and ethical judgment. Such training will enable healthcare managers and professionals to assimilate an organizational culture for promoting an organizational ethical code (Messikomer & Cirka, 2010, p. 60; Shadi et al., 2024).

In 2017 the Geneva Declaration of the World Medical Association (WMA) was updated to meet environmental, internal, and personal changes in how healthcare professionals should be perceived. Codes pertaining to the issue of how to ensure the welfare of healthcare professionals and the nature of their associations with colleagues were also expanded. The processes of change described in this chapter have accelerated in recent years and are expected to become more extreme in the future (McBride et al., 2018), further emphasizing the need to promote medical ethics awareness and ethical judgment among healthcare professionals (Robichaux et al., 2022).

Bioethics, Medical Ethics and Ethical Judgment

The field of bioethics considers ethical questions and issues in the life sciences and medicine, primarily attempting to set limitations and solve problems while establishing and applying social and moral values (Weizman, 2014, p. 14). Medical ethics, a sub-field of bioethics, deals with issues connected to medicine and treatment, such as patient-caregiver relations, euthanasia, abortion, treatment and budget priorities, organ transplants, individual autonomy during treatment, and experimentation with animals and humans.

The field of medical ethics is governed by four guidelines: patient benefits, patient rights to autonomy, refraining from harming patients (even if such harm might benefit and protect society), and justice in the form of equal distribution of health resources. Ethical judgment is defined as the ability to explain and determine which actions, behaviors or approaches are most suitable in a given situation based upon a prevailing set of shared social and cultural values. Ethical judgment or ethical decision-making is often defined as a deliberative process that reflects knowledge of ethical principles, theories, and codes (McBride et al., 2018; Robichaux, 2012), thus serving as a fundamental decision-making tool for differentiating between what is good and bad, right and wrong, or just and unjust for people, organizations, and society at large.

Professional Ethos

Wise (2012, p. 171) defined "professional ethos" as follows:

> A constant negotiation of recognition between professional and other societal actors, and one's self. This recognition depends upon meeting certain contingent professional expectations and norms, but also concerns 'values': how one recognizes, or constructs, one's practice as 'valuable', both professionally and personally.

Professional ethos is accordingly marked by two types of features: internal features found within each professional individual, and external features embedded in the credo of professional organizations (Alt & Raichel, 2018).

Ethical judgment is a critical skill that enables individuals to choose the best solution while focusing on identifying dilemmas and determining proper modes of action relative to a set of social values and existing alternatives. The definition of professional ethos suggests that various factors are liable to serve as impediments by silencing inner values and thus hindering ethical judgment. When a person's internal values clash with the values of the organizational culture, an internal value conflict can occur (McBride et al., 2018; Wolf et al., 2016). In extreme instances such a conflict can engender moral distress: Despite knowing how to act morally, the individual fails to do so and consequently experiences psychological distress due to this failure to do the right thing (Frennert, 2023; Jameton, 2017). This type of distress increases the risk of burnout among healthcare professionals, causing them to withdraw from patient interaction or ultimately leave the healthcare profession (Grace, 2018; Robichaux et al., 2022).

Studies showed that healthcare professionals can be helped to deal with these impediments to ethical judgment by developing moral courage in the form of "willingness to speak out and do what is right in the face of forces that would lead a person to act in some other way" (Lachman, 2007, p. 131). Moral courage enables individuals to stand up publicly for their own principles (Klaassen, 2012) and can be learned and developed through practice and guidance (Faraco et al., 2022; Hawkins & Morse, 2014).

Ethical Leadership Within Healthcare Organizations

Healthcare organizations must cultivate individuals capable of acting as ethical leaders to address ethical and moral dilemmas. This involves equipping them with the necessary skills and resources to navigate complex ethical situations and creating a culture that fosters ethical behavior and encourages the pursuit of ethical solutions (Naamati-Schneider et al., 2024a, 2024b) Ethical leadership refers to the practice of guiding and influencing others through principles of ethical behavior and decision-making. Ethical leadership is defined as demonstration of norms of suitable behavior through personal behavior and interpersonal relations, and the impact of this behavior upon others by means of two-directional communication and decisions making processes Ethical leadership encompasses the practice of guiding and inspiring others based on principles of ethical behavior and ethical decision-making. Ethical leaders strive to create a workplace culture that is grounded in integrity, honesty and accountability, that prioritizes the well-being and development of its team members, and that fosters an environment of mutual respect, trust and fairness. Ethical leadership is essential in promoting an organization's values and goals, together with social responsibility and the common good (Tourigny et al., 2019).

Promoting an Ethical Climate in Healthcare Organizations

Ethical leadership is considered a key factor in creating an ethical organizational climate (Halvorsen et al., 2023). Indeed, Shin (2012) found a positive connection between ethical leadership and promoting an ethical climate within organizations. Ethical leadership influences workers' attitudes and behavior and is associated with being aware of the organization's code of ethics, being involved in making ethical decisions, promoting an ethical climate within the organization, assuming organizational obligations, and enhancing quality of life at work. An ethical climate reflects workers' shared perceptions regarding the ethical content of policies, regulations, and behavior within the organization. Such a climate affects both decision-making and behavioral responses to ethical dilemmas, which can affect various organizational outcomes (Halvorsen et al., 2023). McMurrian and Matulich (2016) also found that creating communication and trust with customers and stakeholders fostered a positive connection between ethical behavior and performance.

Halvorsen et al. (2023) examined the relationship between ethical management education, employee performance, service orientation, and client orientation. Their findings indicated a positive correlation among these variables, particularly when the organizational climate was both ethical and service-oriented. The study suggests that employees who perceive their leaders as ethical and have received ethical training tend to foster an ethical client-oriented organizational climate. Furthermore, ethical leaders play a role in shaping the organizational climate through their exemplary behavior.

Significance of an Ethical Climate and Ethical Guidelines in Organizations

Numerous studies have found that moral dilemmas and ethical obstacles in the medical profession are associated with worker satisfaction, burnout and fatigue Schaefer and Junges (2014) investigated nurses' perceptions of ethical skills, revealing that all faced ethical challenges, with those confident in their ethical attitudes also confident in managing such dilemmas. The study emphasized that merely understanding ethical issues was not enough; practical coping tools were essential. It highlighted three crucial moral foundations for healthcare professionals: personal values, education, and practice. McBride et al. (2018) explored how nurses in US hospitals view the use of electronic health records (EHRs), which are commonly employed for documentation and decision-making in acute care. The study found that EHRs enhanced service and treatment quality and increased staff satisfaction. Nevertheless, accumulating evidence suggests that medical personnel face difficulties using electronic records, including moral distress (Henry et al., 2016; Naamati-Schneider et al., 2024) and challenges surrounding ethical issues that require ethical decision-making models (McBride et al., 2018).

A growing consensus of healthcare professionals contend that a well-defined and digitally compatible ethical framework that is suitable to the digital changes that provide ethical guidelines for healthcare professionals, managers, and medical staff. Such a framework will offer support for medical staff responsible for mediating the many required changes. It will also encompass technology assimilation and the ethical and moral aspects of dealing with technology (McBride et al., 2018). In addition, healthcare professionals are becoming increasingly aware of the need for developing ethical leadership among individuals in the organization.

Numerous scholars have called for passing legislation and establishing legal frameworks concerning this issue. Nevertheless, very few studies have focused on the development of ethical judgment among healthcare system managers. Moreover, there has been limited discussion of the importance of cultivating these skills in the early phases of management education in order to foster ethical judgment capabilities and values. Teaching managers throughout the healthcare system and its organizations to assimilate and develop ethical judgment will help establish internal norms and behavior, thus fostering trust between all players in the system, including patients, and augmenting values of equality within the healthcare system.

Ethical and Ethical Leadership Education

The aim of ethical education is to help students develop new insights about how to live in society and to instill them with a sense of moral obligation. Such education entails presenting and discussing moral philosophies that describe a "good" and "proper" way of life (Ryan & Bisson, 2011). Many studies have considered whether and how to develop and teach ethics and how to cope with environmental issues that are often connected to social beliefs and norms.

Indeed, the importance of ethical education cannot be overemphasized. As early as 2007, the deans of many business management schools cited ethics as their leading objective (Brandenberger & Bowman, 2015; Fan et al., 2022; Orchard, 2021). Other studies have underscored the importance of ethics in education, while at the same time pointing to significant differences in this field. These studies also discussed the problematic nature of ethical education stemming from the numerous challenges in its development and assimilation among students (Laabs, 2012; Vynckier et al., 2015). According to Ryan and Bisson (2011), ethical education can be thought of in terms of a set of rules and principles based on a legal system. Nevertheless, ethics can and should be taught as a set of skills that can be applied. These researchers contended that ethical education is an important communicative process that provides room for social reality and enriches life. Despite the large number of academic courses on ethics, research still indicates that insufficient attention is directed at this topic and that these courses are not taken seriously (Ryan & Bisson, 2011).

Moreover, researchers hold contradictory opinions regarding the effectiveness of ethical education in institutions of higher education. For example, several studies showed that ethical education led to significant improvement in students' ethical attitudes (Ryan & Bisson, 2011), supporting previous studies showing that ethical education improved moral reasoning and increased awareness of and sensitivity to social issues (Stead & Miller, 1988). In contrast, other studies revealed a negative connection between ethical education and students' attitudes (Stephens & Stephens, 2008).

These discussions raise questions about whether ethics should be taught in separate courses or incorporated in all courses within a particular discipline. Some researchers (Ritter, 2006), for example, contend that designated courses are liable to be detached from practical professional repercussions. For students to embrace ethical thinking, they must be taught to assimilate the ethical issues that emerge in various courses.

The multifaceted nature of this problem makes it difficult to offer an unequivocal solution. Integrating ethical content into designated courses can be a potential solution for effectively developing these abilities. Indeed, any proposed curriculum for teaching ethics will undoubtedly help professionals and students understand this complex issue in more depth (Ryan & Bisson, 2011). Effective evaluation and assessment of such programs may be problematic since determining whether students in general courses have indeed assimilated ethical thinking and principles may prove to be difficult. Self-reporting, instructors' reporting, and examining the variables over time as students continue their work in the field can constitute further assessment problems. Moreover, the point of origin of each student must be taken into consideration to determine differential improvement (Berkovich & Eyal, 2020).

Fostering Ethical Behavior: Educational Practices

Due to the importance and multidisciplinary nature of ethics in healthcare, higher education institutions have begun adopting various educational programs aimed at promoting ethical practices and ethical judgment. In the following section, we examine several examples of ethical educational practices, both in specific health professions and in general disciplines. The examples use the Ethical Perspective Instrument (EPI) tool and the Values and Knowledge Education (VaKE) approach (Weyringer et al., 2022).

Berkovich and Eyal (2020) studied the development of ethical judgment among students enrolled in a designated course on ethics. The course was based on several ethical paradigms in conjunction with similar pedagogies that included group discussions and reflection. The researchers measured the students' moral judgment using the EPI (Ethical Perspective Instrument) tool for ethical and moral perception (Eyal et al., 2011). According to the study model, students examined moral dilemmas from each of the following perspectives: *ethics of fairness*—focusing on fair relations; e*thics of utilitarianism*—focusing on optimal benefit; *ethics of concern*—focusing on trust; *ethics of professionalism*—focusing on applying knowledge and professional experience, trust and empowerment in relations; and *community ethics*—focusing upon the interests and values of the community. This extensive form of observation enabled the students to formulate moral codes, promoted their future ethical judgment, and encouraged the best possible solution to any given situation (Shapiro & Stefkovich, 2016).

In this study Shapiro and Stefkovich (2016) claimed that university programs can influence students' moral judgment by fostering their understanding of several ethical perspectives. Carefully constructed ethical education can produce effects that are connected to ethics among a significant number (more than half) of the students. Their results also showed that the type of students initially selected to participate in ethical education greatly influences the effectiveness of their training.

In addition, national and local governments often cooperate with academic programs in an attempt to promote professional codes that shape desired attitudes. These types of initiatives are liable to generate conflicts and antagonism among students, who may sense that attempts are being made to change their attitudes (Berkovich & Eyal, 2020). Other researchers criticized principle-based approaches to ethics education, among other things due to the difficulty of converting abstract material into practical field situations (e.g., complex patient-caregiver relationships) (Hoskins et al., 2018; Pariseau-Legault & Lallier, 2016).

Values and Knowledge Education (VaKE) is another approach to teaching ethics, as assessed in several studies (Alt et al., 2022; Weyringer et al., 2022). VaKE is a useful teaching tool that combines ethics with values-oriented education and content-knowledge education, with emphasis on social behavior and the development of critical thinking in a PBL environment. VaKE suggests using a combination of knowledge and educational aspects to teach a specific field of knowledge and to understand the relationships between theory and practice. Accordingly, the educational process includes dialogue about relevant moral dilemmas. This approach to learning is linked to actual improvement in knowledge, efficacy, skills, resources, and opportunities. It facilitates more effective actions and interpersonal relationships and strives to empower learners.

VaKE incorporates a number of approaches identified with the constructivist approach to learning (Weyringer et al., 2022): cognitive learning, moral development theory and dilemma discussion, and the construction of moral reasoning schemes. Coping with a dilemma entails teamwork and discussing problem-solving alternatives, while considering value aspects and finding relevant information for arguments. This practice is based on exchanging opinions and understanding through listening to others. It focuses on conflicts that engage students in discussion and encourage them to offer conflicting opinions. This approach exposes students to topics relevant to their profession, clarifies the value-related importance of these topics, and allows students to form independent opinions while engaging in dialogue. Indeed, the road to finding a solution may begin with peer dialogue about ethical dilemmas (Alt & Raichel, 2018).

Ethical Education and Ethical Leadership Education in the Healthcare Profession

Despite the lack of consensus regarding what constitutes optimal ethical medical education, various innovative programs have begun to emerge for imparting medical ethics within academic and clinical environments. In the following section, we explore several programs for ethical education and ethical leadership that have been implemented in undergraduate health programs at higher education institutions using team-based learning, student-led learning, and simulation-based learning. Additionally, we discuss ethical education programs for health professionals in clinical settings.

Hickman and Wocial (2013), for example, adopted an active learner approach while integrating team-based learning concepts in an applied ethics course for undergraduate students. The students worked in teams on case-based exercises. The researchers found an increase in participants' moral perception, judgment, and behavior through their mastery of course concepts, team discussions, reflective analysis, and participation in ethical decision-making) Hickkman & Wocial, 2013).

Krautscheid (2017) reported that exposure to scenario simulations helped undergraduate students in surgery courses assimilate ethical dilemmas. During the simulations the students dealt with issues of infection control, treatment safety, and medical confidentiality. Krautscheid found that students gained confidence and improved their preparation and advocacy skills by transferring embedded dilemmas from academia to clinical practice.

Another example is the study by Ford et al. (2024), which investigates the use of "brave spaces" in nursing ethics education. This research focuses on how a structured self-assessment tool, the Engagement Self-Assessment (ESA), affects the development of these spaces in a nursing ethics course. This study highlights the role of supportive educational environments in fostering moral courage and effective handling of ethical issues in healthcare.

Naamati-Schneider and Meirovich (2020, 2022) developed a curriculum that used simulations and ethical dilemmas for instilling values and knowledge in a course that deals with specific dilemmas in patient-caregiver relationships. The course was based entirely on dilemmas and case studies concerning the following topics: violence in the healthcare system, boundaries and exceeding boundaries during treatment, communication in patient-caregiver relationships, trust, and empathy. The instruction method was based on teaching ethical and moral dilemmas using the Student Guided Learning methodology, according to which students direct the learning process. Students must submit a final project in which they examine and present a dilemma from three different standpoints: caregiver, patient, and organization. This three-way examination provides a broad, holistic managerial view that mimics how dilemmas are dealt with in the field, thus enabling students to develop the ability to view a dilemma from different points of view.

Several programs (e.g., APRNS—Advanced Practice Registered Nurses) focus on ethical education at later stages. Pariseau-Legault and Lallier (2016) devised a six-stage ethical framework for making decisions: ethical sensitivity and reflective competence, factual evaluation of the situation, identification of applicable principles, development of deliberative competencies, and evaluation of process outcomes.

Several programs are also offered in clinical frameworks. For example, Grace et al. (2014) developed a special program in ethics at an academic medical center aimed at increasing trust during ethical decision-making. Their goal was to decrease moral distress and train staff members as ethical leaders of change in their field. The program incorporated a variety of pedagogical approaches that served as a basis for moral thinking according to the model developed by Robinson et al. (2014). The model included simulation, didactics, and a mentored clinical practicum. The participants reported increased ethics knowledge, decreased moral distress, and more effective moral agency in clinical practice.

A Global Glance at Ethical Education

As noted, the topic of medical ethics is gaining interest across the globe. For example, nursing and medical students in Japan are required to take a course in professional ethics, and all health profession graduates in Australia must undergo ethics-based competency training (Robichaux et al., 2022). Taiwan and Korea have also called for developing ethical literacy and ethical judgment through ethical education that includes learning problem-based techniques, making correct moral decisions, and engaging in group discussions (Kim & Park, 2019; Lee et al., 2017). Japan in recent years has also begun to be established ethical education frames. In addition to healthcare ethics consultation (HCEC) and assimilation of ethical education in medical academic institutions, a Clinical Ethics Consortium has been launched to provide a forum where those responsible for HCEC in clinical settings can collaborate, exchange information, and conduct discussions (Nagao & Takimoto, 2023). Educators in the fields of nursing, health management, and medicine face similar problems, and they often have difficulty determining specific objectives or agreeing on definitions and effectiveness in this field (Chen, 2023; Robichaux et al., 2022). Empirical data are limited and there is a discrepancy between what is taught in academia and what occurs in clinical healthcare practice, with local practices prevailing in all professional areas at all stages of training (Hoskins et al., 2018; Laabs, 2015).

Today researchers are being called upon to expand research and knowledge in the area of clinical, medical and managerial education to better prepare healthcare staff and managers for ethical practice and management in the field. Ethical education must be broad and uniform so as to create a suitable environment that can constitute a managerial and ethical treatment framework for healthcare professionals. Additional research is clearly needed to assess the critical role played by ethical education in coping with patient treatment quality, health equality problems, interdisciplinary cooperation, and healthcare professionals' satisfaction and overall health. Studies examining methodologies for developing moral leadership and moral judgment should be expanded, and moral courage must be augmented to alleviate moral distress (Ulrich, 2015).

Moreover, while the various players in the healthcare realm (e.g., doctors, nurses, and managers) each must cope with specific issues, there is extensive overlap between them, necessitating the establishment of a shared interdisciplinary foundation of ethical knowledge to benefit caregivers, patients, and the system as a whole. Collaboration is needed to build the core components of ethical education, along with research to assess the impact of ethical teaching on patients and healthcare professionals (Chen, 2023; Hoskins et al., 2018).

Promoting Ethical Standards and Values Globally Through Uniform Programs

Attempts are also underway to generate uniform reports and programs in the field of medical ethics. The authors of the 2015 Romanell Report, for example, proposed clear-cut goals and objectives in an attempt to create a document for ethics educators that sets out desired ethical objectives together with instruction methods and strategies for assimilating them. The report specifically discussed assimilating ethical principles or combining them with a study program that emphasizes the benefits of various pedagogical methods. It also recommended using assessment methods to connect medical ethics and professionalism education with patient outcomes (Carrese, 2015).

The American Association of Colleges of Nursing (AACN) made another such attempt by proposing the formation of committees to review and update ethical requirements at all levels: Core Competencies for Professional Nursing Education (AACN, 2021).

Another universal and extensive UNESCO project focuses on bioethics through the Bioethics Core Curriculum Program. This program offers a defined structure covering many topics that are further divided into units. It includes an ethical method for analyzing situations and dilemmas that can be used to investigate incidents according to several steps: fact deliberation, value deliberation, duty deliberation, consistency testing, and final decision. The program also offers comprehensive learning materials, articles, films, and academic materials for lecturers and instructors (UNESCO, 2016). Jegan and Dierickx (2023) attempted to assess the degree to which such global programs have been adopted. They found that value-based guidelines tend to be more globally applicable than norm-based guidelines, which tend to be more context-specific and thus to differ from country to country. Despite contradictory opinions regarding teaching mode and technology use, scholars nevertheless agree on the importance of this topic and its assimilation among both healthcare providers and managers at all levels of the healthcare system. The need to move from traditional instruction methods to a competence-based education is becoming widely accepted (Sistermans, 2020).

In June 2017, the Macy Foundation asked educators in the healthcare professions to review the current state of competency-based professional health education. The group made the following recommendations regarding health ethics: redesign curricula to achieve a successful, competency-based education system in the health professions; create a continuum of education, training, practice and assessment; enable the use of technologies in implementing competency-based-education throughout the education continuum (Josiah Macy Jr. Foundation, 2017). Although these recommendations are not specific to the field of ethics, they provide a suitable framework for integrating interdisciplinary models that focus on translating and implementing theoretical knowledge in the field and in clinical practice. Additional research is clearly needed to develop these areas (Chen, 2023; Hoskins et al., 2018; Robichaux et al., 2022).

Discussion

The broad consensus today is that managers in the healthcare system must adapt to a complex changing environment in order to function on a daily basis. The development of ethical medical education and attitudes and the formation of a leadership identity are essential for achieving this objective. Healthcare system directors must make managerial and treatment decisions every day, while at the same time making moral and ethical judgments within the legal framework (e.g., resource allotment, medical research ethics, public health policies, more). Programs offering ethical education have become an inseparable part of the training provided for medical personnel (Robichaux et al., 2022). The consensus is that there is no single effective pedagogical strategy. Consequently, a number of different strategies should be employed throughout professional training as well as during clinical and managerial work in the field (Lee et al., 2020).

In addition to the consistent need for programs using various methodologies, and despite the extent of these activities across the globe, they still need to be assimilated across all healthcare professions. The vast number of global programs reflects the numerous changes in the field and the perception that these processes are essential. Attempts are being made to attain formal certification for these programs and to establish official regulations and standards.

This chapter has underscored the fundamental need for ethical education, beginning with training for working in medical professions and continuing during field practice. The necessarily solution will likely involve changing systematic paradigms together with adopting an organizational focus that is ethically oriented. System-wide planning and budgeting will facilitate the creation of "ethics management centers" within organizations that will be responsible for ongoing development and training in these issues in all health professions and disciplines. Ethical education will be required for all health system workers, with emphasis on managers so as to achieve better control over ethical education (Nagao & Takimoto, 2023).

These centers will be responsible for coordinating in-service training courses and ongoing training to further develop the necessary skills. They will coordinate with academia to establish ongoing courses for beginning students and provide practical support. They will also create a uniform ethical language that will facilitate ethical dialogue and the development of ethical knowledge and capabilities among all healthcare professionals. Providing ethical education for all staff members, regardless of gender, culture or role, will offer diverse perspectives and may facilitate the resolution of ethical dilemmas.

The proposed framework can also act as a foundation for intra-organizational communication. It can promote consolidation of these programs and facilitate lateral integration of such processes across multiple countries, using a common language. This integration should also yield joint research with emphasis placed on developing research and clinical practice throughout the healthcare system.

References

Allen, M. R., Webb, S., Mandvi, A., Frieden, M., Tai-Seale, M., & Kallenberg, G. (2024). Navigating the doctor-patient-AI relationship-a mixed-methods study of physician attitudes toward artificial intelligence in primary care. *BMC Primary Care, 25*(1), 42. https://doi.org/10.1186/s12875-024-02282-y

Alt, D., & Raichel, N. (2018). *Lifelong citizenship: Lifelong learning as a lever for moral and democratic values*. Brill and Sense Publishers.

Alt, D., Weinberger, A., Heinrichs, K., & Naamati-Schneider, L. (2022). The role of goal orientations and learning approaches in explaining digital concept mapping utilization in problem-based learning. *Current Psychology*, 1–16. https://doi.org/10.1007/s12144-021-02613-7

American Association of Colleges of Nursing. (2021). *The essentials: Core competencies for professional nursing education*. AACN-Essentials. https://www.aacnnursing.org/

Berkovich, I., & Eyal, O. (2020). Ethics education in leadership development: Adopting multiple ethical paradigms. *Educational Management Administration & Leadership, 48*(2), 270–285. https://doi.org/10.1177/1741143218792914

Brandenberger, J. W., & Bowman, N. A. (2015). Prosocial growth during college: Results of a national study. *Journal of Moral Education, 44*(3), 328–345. https://doi.org/10.1080/03057240.2015.1048792

Carrese, J. A., Malek, J., Watson, K., Lehmann, L. S., Green, M. J., McCullough, L. B., Geller, G., Braddock, C. H., & Doukas, D. J. (2015). The essential role of medical ethics education in achieving professionalism: The Romanell report. *Academic Medicine: Journal of the Association of American Medical Colleges, 90*(6), 744–752. https://doi.org/10.1377/hlthaff.2014.0128

Chen, L. (2023). Analysis of the problems and countermeasures of medical ethics education in medical schools. *Contemporary Education and Teaching Research, 4*(1), 5–8. https://doi.org/10.47852/bonviewCETR2023040102

Dean, W., Talbot, S., & Dean, A. (2019). Reframing clinician distress: Moral injury not burnout. *Federal Practitioner, 36*(9), 400–402. https://doi.org/10.1590/S0080-6234201400002000019

Eyal, O., Berkovich, I., & Schwartz, T. (2011). Making the right choice: Ethical judgments among educational leaders. *Journal of Educational Administration, 49*(4), 396–413. https://doi.org/10.1108/09578231111146470

Fan, X., Johnson, R., Liu, X., & Gao, R. (2022). College students' views of ethical issues in classroom assessment in Chinese higher education. *Studies in Higher Education, 47*(1), 131–145.

Faraco, M. M., Gelbcke, F. L., Brehmer, L. C. D. F., et al. (2022). Moral distress and moral resilience of nurse managers. *Nursing Ethics, 29*(5), 1253–1265. https://doi.org/10.1177/09697330221085770

Fenton, J. J., Jerant, A. F., Bertakis, K. D., & Franks, P. (2012). The cost of satisfaction: A national study of patient satisfaction, health care utilization, expenditures, and mortality. *Archives of Internal Medicine, 172*(5), 405–411. https://doi.org/10.1001/archinternmed.2011.1662

Ford, N. J., Gomes, L. M., & Brown, S. B. (2024). Brave spaces in nursing ethics education: Courage through pedagogy. *Nursing Ethics, 31*(1), 101–113. https://doi.org/10.1177/09697330231183075

Frennert, S. (2023). Moral distress and ethical decision-making of eldercare professionals involved in digital service transformation. *Disability and Rehabilitation. Assistive Technology, 18*(2), 156–165. https://doi.org/10.1080/17483107.2020.1839579

Grace, P., Robinson, E., Jurchak, M., Zollfrank, A., & Lee, S. (2014). Clinical ethics residency for nurses: An education model to decrease moral distress and strengthen nurse retention in acute care. JONA: *The Journal of Nursing Administration, 44*(12), 640–646. https://doi.org/10.1097/NNA.0000000000000141

Grace, P. (2018). Enhancing nurse moral agency: The leadership promise of doctor of nursing practice preparation. *Online Journal of Issues in Nursing, 23*(1). https://doi.org/10.3912/OJIN.Vol23No01Man04

Hall, M. A., Bobinski, M. A., Orentlicher, D., Cohen, I. G., Bagley, N., & Sawicki, N. N. (2024). *Health care law and ethics*. Aspen Publishing

Halvorsen, B., Bartram, T., Kia, N., & Cavanagh, J. (2023). Meeting customer needs through ethical leadership and training: Examining Australian bank employees. *Asia Pacific Journal of Human Resources, 61*(1), 79–100. https://doi.org/10.1111/1744-7941.12329

Hawkins, S. F., & Morse, J. (2014). The praxis of courage as a foundation for care. *Journal of Nursing Scholarship*, 46(4), 263–270. https://doi.org/10.1111/jnu.12077

Henry, J., Pylypchuk, Y., Searcy, T., & Patel, V. (2016). *Adoption of electronic health record systems among U.S. non-federal acute care hospitals: 2008–2015*. Office of National Coordinator for Health IT. Retrieved from https://dashboard.healthit.gov/evaluations/data-briefs/non-federal-acute-care-hospital-ehradoption-2008-2015

Hickman, S. E., & Wocial, L. D. (2013). Team-based learning and ethics education in nursing. *The Journal of Nursing Education, 52*(12), 696–700. https://doi.org/10.3928/01484834-20131121-01

Hoskins, K., Grady, C., & Ulrich, C. M. (2018). Ethics education in nursing: Instruction for future generations of nurses. *The Online Journal of Issues in Nursing*, 23(1), Manuscript 3. https://doi.org/10.3912/OJIN.Vol23No01Man03

Ijiga, A. C., Peace, A. E., Idoko, I. P., Agbo, D. O., Harry, K. D., Ezebuka, C. I., & Ukatu, I. E. (2024). Ethical considerations in implementing generative AI for healthcare supply chain optimization: A cross-country analysis across India, the United Kingdom, and the United States of America. *International Journal of Biological and Pharmaceutical Sciences Archive, 7*(01), https://doi.org/10.53771/ijbpsa.2024.7.1.0015

Jameton, A. (2017). What moral distress in nursing history could suggest about the future of health care. *AMA Journal of Ethics, 19*(6), 617–628. https://doi.org/10.1001/journalofethics.2017.19.6.mhst1-1706

Jegan, R., & Dierickx, K. (2023). Ethics without borders: An analysis of national and international guidelines on ethics in basic medical education. *Advances in Health Sciences Education*, 1-22. https://doi.org/10.1007/s10459-022-10186-8

Josiah Macy Jr. Foundation. (2017). *Achieving competency-based, time-variable health professions education*. Retrieved from http://macyfoundation.org/publications/publication/conference-summary-achieving-competency-based-time-variable-education

Karni, T., & Reches, A. (2018). *The ethics board rules and position papers*. Israeli Medical Association.

Khosravi, M., Zare, Z., Mojtabaeian, S. M., & Izadi, R. (2024). Ethical challenges of using artificial intelligence in healthcare delivery: A thematic analysis of a systematic review of reviews. *Journal of Public Health*, 1–11. https://doi.org/10.1007/s10389-024-02219-w

Kim, W. J., & Park, J. H. (2019). The effects of debate-based ethics education on the moral sensitivity and judgment of nursing students: A quasi-experimental study. *Nurse Education Today, 83*, 104200. https://doi.org/10.1016/j.nedt.2019.08.018. PMID:31491613.

Klaassen, C. (2012). Just a teacher or also a moral example? In D. Alt & R. Reingold (Eds.), *Changes in teachers' moral role. From passive observers to moral and democratic leaders* (pp. 13–30). Sense.

Krautscheid, L. C. (2017). Embedding microethical dilemmas in high-fidelity simulation scenarios: Preparing nursing students for ethical practice. *The Journal of Nursing Education, 56*(1), 55–58. https://doi.org/10.3928/01484834-20161219-11

Laabs, C. A. (2012). Confidence and knowledge regarding ethics among advanced practice nurses. *Nursing Education Perspectives, 33*(1), 10–14. https://doi.org/10.5480/1536-5026-33.1.10.

Laabs, C. A. (2015). Toward a consensus in ethics education for the doctor of nursing practice. *Nursing Education Perspectives, 36*(4), 249–251. https://doi.org/10.5480/13-1195

Lachman, V. D. (2007). Moral courage in action: Case studies. *Medsurg Nursing: Official Journal of the Academy of Medical-Surgical Nurses, 16*(4), 275. Retrieved from http://www.ncbi.nlm.nih.gov/pubmed/17907703

Lee, H. L., Huang, S. H., & Huang, C. M. (2017). Evaluating the effect of three teaching strategies on student nurses' moral sensitivity. *Nursing Ethics, 24*(6), 732–743. https://doi.org/10.1177/0969733015623095. PMID:26822297.

Lee, S., Robinson, E. M., Grace, P. J., Zollfrank, A., & Jurchak, M. (2020). Developing a moral compass: Themes from the clinical ethics residency for nurses (CERN) final essays. *Nursing Ethics, 27*(1), 28–39. https://doi.org/10.1177/0969733019833125

Martell, K. (2007). Assessing student learning: Are business schools making the grade? *Journal of Education for Business, 82*(4), 189–196. https://doi.org/10.3200/JOEB.82.4.189-195

McMurrian, R. C., & Matulich, E. (2016). Building customer value and profitability with business ethics. *Journal of Business & Economics Research (JBER), 14*(3), 83–90. https://doi.org/10.19030/jber.v14i3.9748

McBride, S., Tietze, M., Hanley, M. A., & Thomas, L. (2017). Statewide study to assess nurses' experiences with meaningful use-based electronic health records. *Computers, Informatics, Nursing, 35*(1), 18–28. https://doi.org/10.1097/CIN.0000000000000290

McBride, S., Tietze, M., Hanley, M. A., & Thomas, L. (2015). *Statewide study assessing the experience of nurses with their electronic health records.* Texas Nurses Association. Retrieved from https://c.ymcdn.com/sites/www.texasnurses.org/resource/resmgr/HIT_Files/HIT_Survey_Report-Final.pdf

McBride, S., Tietze, M., Robichaux, C., Stokes, L., & Weber, E. (2018). Identifying and addressing ethical issues with use of electronic health records. *OJIN: The Online Journal of Issues in Nursing, 23*(1), Manuscript 5. https://doi.org/10.3912/OJIN.Vol23No01Man05

Messikomer, C. M., & Cirka, C. C. (2010). Constructing a code of ethics: An experiential case of a national professional organization. *Journal of Business Ethics*, 95(1), 55–71. https://doi.org/10.1007/s10551-009-0347-y

Naamati Schneider, L., & Meirovich, A. (2020). Student guided learning-from teaching to e-learning. *Romanian Journal for Multidimensional Education/Revista Romaneasca pentru Educatie Multidimensionala, 12.* 115–121. https://doi.org/10.18662/rrem/12.1sup2/254

Naamati-Schneider, L. (2021). Public-private: Unequal competition: Israeli public hospitals versus the private healthcare system following government reforms. *International Journal of Organisational Analysis, 29*(6), 1381–1394. https://doi.org/10.1108/IJOA-06-2020-2237

Naamati-Schneider, L. (2022). Intra-organisation conflicts of interest in hospitals adapting to a changing ecosystem. *Journal of Health Organisation and Management, 36*(3), 265–278. https://doi.org/10.1108/JHOM-09-2021-0325

Naamati-Schneider, L., & Meirovich, A. (2022). Students guided learning for medical students: Novel teaching for the 21st century. In *Medical education for the 21st century* (p. 77). IntechOpen. https://doi.org/10.5772/intechopen.98823

Naamati-Schneider, L., & Zaks, O. (2022). Public hospitals in crisis: Managerial and strategic adaptation. In D. Vrontis, A. Thrassou, Y. Weber, S. M. R. Shams, E. Tsoukatos, & L. Efthymiou (Eds.), *Business under crisis, Volume II. Palgrave studies in cross-disciplinary business research.* In Association with EuroMed Academy of Business. Palgrave Macmillan. https://doi.org/10.1007/978-3-030-76575-0_3

Naamati-Schneider L, Arazi-Fadlon M, Daphna-Tekoah S. (2024a). Strategic technological processes in hospitals: Conflicts and personal experiences of healthcare teams. *Nursing Ethics* 0(0). https://doi.org/10.1177/09697330241252876

Naamati-Schneider, L., Arazi-Fadlon M., & Daphna-Tekoah, S. (2024b). Navigating moral and ethical dilemmas and conflict in strategic technological processes within healthcare organizations. *Digital Health.*

Naamati-Schneider, L. (2023). The effect of digitalization on service orientation and service perception among Israeli healthcare professionals: A qualitative study. *Digital Health, 9.* https://doi.org/10.1177/20552076231191892

Nagao, N., & Takimoto, Y. (2023). Clinical ethics consultation in Japan: What does it mean to have a functioning ethics consultation? https://doi.org/10.21203/rs.3.rs-2375779/v1

Olorunsogo, T., Adenyi, A. O., Okolo, C. A., & Babawarun, O. (2024). Ethical considerations in AI-enhanced medical decision support systems: A review. *World Journal of Advanced Engineering Technology and Sciences, 11*(1), 329–336. https://doi.org/10.30574/wjaets.2024.11.1.0061

Orchard, J. (2021). Moral education and the challenge of pre-service professional formation for teachers. *Journal of Moral Education, 50*(1), 104–113. https://doi.org/10.1080/03057240.2020.1763932

Pariseau-Legault, P., & Lallier, M. (2016). Constructing an ethical training for advanced nursing practice: An interactionist and competency-based approach. *The Journal of Nursing Education, 55*(7), 399–402. https://doi.org/10.3928/01484834-20160615-08

Powers, T. L., & Bendall, D. (2004). Improving health outcomes through patient empowerment. *Journal of Hospital Marketing & Public Relations, 15*(1), 45–59. https://doi.org/10.2139/ssrn.2140763

Präg, P., Wittek, R., & Mills, M. (2017). The educational gradient in self-rated health in Europe: Does the doctor–patient relationship make a difference? *Acta Sociologica, 60*(4), 325–341. https://doi.org/10.1177/0001699316670715

Rathert, C., Mittler, J. N., Banerjee, S., & McDaniel, J. (2016). Patient-centered communication in the era of electronic health records: What does the evidence say? *Patient Education and Counseling, 100*(1), 50–64. https://doi.org/10.1016/j.pec.2016.07.031

Ritter, B. A. (2006). Can business ethics be trained? A study of the ethical decision-making process in business students. *Journal of Business Ethics, 68*, 153–164.

Robichaux, C. (2012). Developing ethical skills: From sensitivity to action. *Critical Care Nurse, 32*(2), 65–72. https://doi.org/10.4037/ccn2012929

Robichaux, C., Grace, P., Bartlett, J., Stokes, F., Saulo Lewis, M., & Turner, M. (2022). Ethics education for nurses: Foundations for an integrated curriculum. *The Journal of Nursing Education, 61*(3), 123–130. https://doi.org/10.3928/01484834-20220109-02

Robinson, E. M., Lee, S. M., Zollfrank, A., Jurchak, M., Frost, D., & Grace, P. (2014). Enhancing moral agency: Clinical ethics residency for nurses. *Hastings Center Report, 44*(5), 12–20. https://doi.org/10.1002/hast.353

Ryan, T. G., & Bisson, J. (2011). Can ethics be taught? *International Journal of Business and Social Science*, 2(12). https://doi.org/10.1038/273579a0

Schaefer, R., & Junges, J. R. (2014). The construction of ethical competence in the perception of primary care nurses. *Revista da Escola de Enfermagem da USP, 48*, 329–334.

Shadi, A. Z., Zohreh, V., Eesa, M., & Anoshirvan, K. (2024). Moral sensitivity of nursing students: A systematic review. *BMC Nursing, 23*(1), 99. https://doi.org/10.1186/s12912-024-01713-6

Shapiro, J., & Stefkovich, J. A. (2016). *Ethical leadership and decision making in education: Applying theoretical perspectives to complex dilemmas* (4th ed.). Routledge. https://doi.org/10.4324/9781315773339

Shin, Y. (2012). CEO ethical leadership, ethical climate, climate strength, and collective organizational citizenship behavior. *Journal of Business Ethics, 108*(3), 299–312. https://doi.org/10.1007/s10551-011-1091-7

Sistermans, I. J. (2020). Integrating competency-based education with a case-based or problem-based learning approach in online health sciences. *Asia Pacific Education Review, 21*(4), 683–696.

Stead, B. A., & Miller, J. J. (1988). Can social awareness be increased through business school curricula. *Journal of Business Ethics, 7*, 553–560.

Stephens, V. R., & Stephens, A. S. (2008). An examination of accounting majors' ethical decisions before and after an ethics course requirement. *Journal of College Teaching & Learning*, 5 (4) 49–55. https://doi.org/10.19030/tlc.v5i4.1278

Sulmasy, L., López, A., & Horwitch, C. (2017). Ethical implications of the electronic health record: In the service of the patient. *Journal of General Internal Medicine, 32*(8), 935–939. https://doi.org/10.1007/s11606-017-4030-1

Tekkeşin, A. İ. (2019). Artificial intelligence in healthcare. *Anatolian Journal of Cardiology, 22*(1), 8–9. https://doi.org/10.14744/AnatolJCardiol.2019.28

TerKonda, S. P., & Fish, E. M. (2023). Artificial intelligence viewed through the lens of state regulation. *Intelligence-Based Medicine, 100088*. https://doi.org/10.1016/j.ibmed.2023.100088

Tourigny, L., Han, J., Baba, V. V., & Pan, P. (2019). Ethical leadership and corporate social responsibility in China: A multilevel study of their effects on trust and organizational citizenship behavior. *Journal of Business Ethics, 158*, 427–440.

UNESCO. (2016). Bioethics core curriculum, section 1: Syllabus Ethics Education Programme (Document code: SHS-2016/WS/12). https://unesdoc.unesco.org/ark:/48223/pf0000244957

Ulrich, C. (2015). Goals of and approaches to bioethics education. Presentation to the Presidential Commission for the Study of Bioethical Issues, May 27. Retrieved from http://bioethics.gov/node/4945

Vynckier, T., Gastmans, C., Cannaerts, N., & de Casterle, B. D. (2015). Effectiveness of ethics education as perceived by nursing students: Development and testing of a novel assessment instrument. *Nursing Ethics, 22*(3), 287–306. https://doi.org/10.1177/0969733014538887

Weizman, R. (2021). *50 dilemmas in medical ethics*. Niv Books. (In Hebrew)

Weyringer, S., Patry, J. L., Pnevmatikos, D., & Børhaug, F. B. (2022). *The VaKE handbook: Theory and practice of values and knowledge education* (Vol. 18). Brill.

Wise, S. (2012). Working to think otherwise: Tracing ethos in information professionals' reflections on learning and practice. *Australian Academic & Research Libraries, 43*, 169–188. https://doi.org/10.1080/00048623.2012.10722276

Wolf, L. A., Perhats, C., Delao, A. M., Moon, M. D., Clark, P. R., & Zavotsky, K. E. (2016). It's a burden you carry: Describing moral distress in emergency nursing. *Journal of Emergency Nursing, 42*(1), 37. https://doi.org/10.1016/j.jen.2015.08.008

World Medical Association. (2017). *WMA Declaration of Geneva*. Retrieved from https://www.wma.net/policies-post/wma-declaration-of-geneva/

Part IV
Interpersonal Competencies

Chapter 9
Managerial Leadership in Healthcare Systems

Abstract Understanding the nuances between medical leadership and management is crucial for the effective functioning of healthcare systems. This chapter explores these differences and overlaps by examining various models and forms of medical leadership and intervention programs. It traces the educational progress of leadership training from students to senior managers, highlighting the evolving dynamics of change within the healthcare system and its managerial leadership. Key educational strategies for fostering effective medical management leadership are identified, emphasizing timely planning, awareness of challenges, and the development of leadership skills. This approach aims to ensure system stability and improve patient care by strategically planning change processes.

Introduction

Healthcare organizations must deal with a broad range of demographic, economic, legal and social changes that characterize the global and local ecosystem in which they operate (discussed in Chap. 2). They must operate within a VUCA World dominated by volatility, uncertainty, complexity and ambiguity (Worley & Jules, 2020). These factors have constant and dramatic repercussions upon how healthcare organizations conduct themselves and function on a daily basis (Senkubuge et al., 2014). The need to cope with market conditions presents numerous challenges in implementing and assimilating extensive changes at all levels of the organization (Cernega et al., 2024; Ginter et al., 2018; Naamati-Schneider, 2020; Naamati-Schneider & Salvatore, 2023). These change processes compel healthcare organizations to adopt various business and management behaviors that are essential for their survival. Yet these behaviors frequently contradict the organization's culture, often requiring broad and comprehensive changes in attitudes, outlooks and values that present many difficulties and challenges. To cope with these challenges, healthcare organizations must assimilate and strengthen the leadership abilities of those in charge of change throughout the system (Figueroa et al., 2019; Naamati-Schneider, 2022, 2023).

L. Naamati-Schneider and D. Alt, *Technology and Competency-Oriented Learning*,
https://doi.org/10.1007/978-981-97-5771-8_9

This chapter defines and discusses the development of the concept of leadership. It reviews various leadership styles and clarifies the differences between traditional management and medical leadership. It demonstrates the importance of adopting leadership capabilities in health systems worldwide and reviews the development, assimilation and evaluation of a variety of programs for fostering leadership in medical education and health organizations. By planning early, understanding anticipated difficulties and developing medical management and leadership capabilities, healthcare organizations can train professional manpower and institute processes of change that will make the system more stable and enable it to provide better service (Figueroa et al., 2019).

Leadership and Management

Definitions of leadership have emerged over time, in accordance with different needs and outlooks. House (1971), for example, defined leadership as the ability to influence, motivate and enable others to act. According to Northouse (2011), leadership is a process in which a group of people act together to attain a common goal. Often the definition of leadership refers to power or energy that creates a vision or direction and helps motivate action (Swanwick & McKimm, 2017). Indeed, leadership is directly connected to influencing and generating change. Consequently, leaders must be influential individuals capable of shaping the behavior, thinking and values of others. They do this through dyadic relationships that enable them to mobilize others and earn their support to achieve common objectives, implement changes and promote an overriding vision (Ahlsson, 2020; Anthony & Huckshorn, 2008; Laverack, 2014; Oates, 2012; Whelehan et al., 2021).

Leadership is currently acknowledged as one of the most significant factors in organizational success and in creating a positive atmosphere and culture (McKimm et al., 2022). Most research in this area has focused on those in managerial positions of authority. Nevertheless, it is important to differentiate between leadership and authority. People in managerial positions do not necessarily identify with the vision and objectives of the organization. Their primary functions are organizational in that they deal with planning, budgeting, control, problem-solving and human resource allocation. Leaders, on the other hand, act based on choice and identification with the organization's vision and objectives regardless of whether they hold managerial positions (Heifetz et al., 2009). Managers exert direct and formal power, whereas leaders make use of informal and indirect power. The job of leaders is to create and lead change, to determine direction and to motivate workers to implement these changes (Van Diggele et al., 2020). People in leadership roles determine the organizational vision, whereas management is responsible for implementing this vision, among other things by identifying problems and finding solutions (McKimm & Jones, 2018). Management provides stability in matters related to finances, academics and human resources so that changes can be implemented without upsetting the overall stability of the organization. According to Bernstein et al. (2016), one way to differentiate between leadership and management is based on function. For example, management is mainly responsible for the organization's reliability, whereas its leadership is responsible for its ability to adapt. Numerous studies have differentiated between the roles, personality characteristics, traits and abilities of leaders and those of managers (Kotter, 2008). In the past, leadership was thought to be an inborn trait that found expression in managerial jobs (Ewens, 2002). Today every person is thought to have the potential for leadership, and this potential can be nurtured and even adapted to specific situations. In recent decades, the notion that leadership can be developed and nurtured has led to the development of different leadership ideologies and styles (McKimm et al., 2022).

Leadership Styles

Scholars have proposed various models of leadership styles. Some of these models emphasize the types of organizations in which leaders work: commercial, educational or military. Others focus on leaders' outlooks and perceptions regarding their jobs, their authority and their relationships with others. In the following sections we examine several of these models.

Rewarding Leadership and Transformational Leadership

According to Burns (2012), leaders who adopt a rewarding style of leadership offer material rewards and punishments in exchange for the work and loyalty of others based on the belief that people work to gain their objectives at any cost. Transformational leaders, on the other hand, establish contact with others while focusing on internal needs as a high priority. These leaders facilitate the development of awareness and new ways of attaining results while creating a sense of mission. Transformational leaders work to attain their goals by using the world of values their followers identify with. This form of leadership stresses the dynamics of motivation by creating internal commitment. Transformative leaders are referred to as such because they are able to encourage workers to make a transition from self–interest to collective interest. Indeed, they generate changes in their followers' ambitions and self-expectations. They no longer compromise or accept the organization's previously accepted norms but rather transform these norms. Transformative leaders help create inner commitment among workers by exercising responsibility, underscoring significance and setting a personal example (Bruce et al., 2019; Swanwick & McKimm, 2017).

Goleman's Leadership Styles

Another leadership style model (Goleman, 2017) is based upon the organization's decision-making style, which is fundamentally influenced by his theoretical work on emotional intelligence. Goleman's theoretical work on emotional intelligence provides the foundation for his leadership style model. Emotional intelligence, which encompasses self-awareness, self-regulation, motivation, empathy, and social skills, is crucial in shaping effective decision-making and leadership practices within organizations. The decision-making style model proposes a management scale comprising six styles: coercive, authoritarian, affiliative, democratic, pacesetting and coaching. These six styles describe different ways in which leaders can interact with and motivate their teams. Each style has its own unique strengths and weaknesses. The coercive style entails a top-down approach in which leaders demand immediate compliance from their team members. The authoritative style involves setting a clear vision and direction for team members while giving them the freedom to achieve this vision in their own way. The affiliative style emphasizes the importance of building relationships and creating a positive work environment. The democratic style involves encouraging participation and input from team members when making decisions. The pacesetting style includes setting high expectations for team members and leading by example. Finally, the coaching style involves focusing on the personal and professional development of team members. Leaders who use the coaching style provide feedback and guidance to help team members improve their skills and achieve their goals.

Effective leaders are able to adapt their style to suit their team and the situation. Understanding the various styles along the management scale can help leaders identify which approach is best suited for different scenarios and cultivate the skills necessary to succeed. Ultimately, effective leadership requires a deep understanding of emotional intelligence and the ability to connect with and motivate team members.

Different styles of leadership can occur simultaneously within an organization. Indeed, leadership styles differ from one person to another and may change according to the personal or organizational environment. Moreover, good leaders who achieve the best results may employ more than one style of leadership. As a result of the radical change processes brought about by the VUCA World during the last decade, many organizations have been forced to change in order to cope and survive in the various markets (Worley & Jules, 2020). These conditions present organizations and their workers with adaptive challenges at all levels of the system and have repercussions on management tasks, necessitating the development of an adaptive leadership style.

Adaptive Leadership

The term adaptive leadership was coined by Heifetz et al. (2009) and is based upon the evolutionary perception that in order to operate it is necessary to adapt to the environment. This type of leadership and management posits that some problems and challenges cannot be solved simply or immediately due to the ecosystem surrounding the organization. For this reason, change and adaptation to the environment require multidisciplinary action and broad cooperation rather than depending upon one person. This type of leadership is based on identifying risks and problems and employing futuristic innovative thinking in problem solving (Choflet et al., 2021; McKimm et al., 2022; Nelson & Squires, 2017). It is therefore characterized by bottom-to-top innovation that brings about extensive and ongoing changes involving staff members at all organizational levels. According to this approach, every individual in the organization can potentially take initiative, play an active role and influence the system.

Adaptive leadership is based on the following four principles: (1) Organizational justice: Leaders create an environment in which every member of the organization can be heard. (2) Emotional intelligence: Adaptive leadership recognizes relationships. (3) Development: Adaptive leaders empower responsibility and encourage learning processes. (4) Character: Adaptive leaders demonstrate ethical responsibility and morals. Hence, adaptive leaders create an environment that enables every member of the organization to be heard, empower their colleagues to learn and grow, and hold themselves accountable to high ethical standards (McKimm et al., 2022).

Holacratic Leadership

Another leadership style that is becoming more and more prevalent in situations and organizations marked by an increasing rate of change and shared processes is holacratic leadership. This concept, introduced by Robertson (2007), refers to an organizational structure characterized by a lack of managerial hierarchy. Instead, it is based on task management within work circles in which all workers jointly strive to achieve the circle's tasks and goals. In the holacratic leadership model, authority is distributed across teams and individuals rather than being concentrated in a hierarchical structure. This approach encourages individuals to take on multiple roles within the organization and work collaboratively to achieve shared goals. Rather than being based on the traditional top-down management structure, decision-making is decentralized and achieved through a transparent process of governance. Overall, holacratic leadership focuses on fostering autonomy, accountability and collaboration among team members while encouraging continuous improvement and innovation in the organization (Mazilu & Dobrescu, 2020).

Leadership in Healthcare

Healthcare organizations must also operate within the VUCA World reality (Worley & Jules, 2020). This reality incorporates specific changes that characterize the healthcare system market and its organizations and affect how healthcare organizations have coped with the complex and extensive challenges of recent decades—challenges stemming from various factors in their local and global environments (Counte et al., 2019; Otter, 2019; WHO, 2016, 2019). These complexities force healthcare systems and organizations to adopt adaptation processes at all levels that necessitate changes in business, marketing, services, management and healthcare (Maeda & Socha-Dietrich, 2021; Naamati-Scineider, 2020).

Medical leadership is therefore essential for effective change management. According to the model for assimilating strategic changes in healthcare organizations proposed by Ginter et al. (2018), change processes occur in stages and encompass all levels of management and workers. In response, organizations must establish a vision, set goals, involve all workers and motivate them to act. Consequently, developing leadership capabilities among healthcare system managers and medical workers is essential for identifying and adapting to existing challenges and reinforcing the system to withstand unstable environmental conditions and intense competition.

The need to develop and empower healthcare leadership is relevant to all three levels of the healthcare system described previously in this book: the macro-system level, the meso-organizational level, and the micro-personal level. Changing needs dictate comprehensive change processes at all levels of the system, necessitating meta-leadership. Horizontal perceptions of system-wide leadership need to be reevaluated during leadership crises such as the COVID-19 pandemic in order to establish a comprehensive picture of change and adaptation to change (Marcus et al., 2015; McKimm et al., 2022).

Developing meta-leadership in the healthcare field is important at the overall macro-system level due to its dramatic effect on entire communities worldwide (McKimm et al., 2022). Medical leadership at the meso-organizational level is needed to understand that adopting change processes requires the cooperation of everyone in the system in dealing with environmental changes. Leading change processes, therefore, requires organizational flexibility, cooperation and transformative leadership that will enable all individuals to adopt change processes while being proactive so that they become capable of leading changes and formulating and assimilating common organizational goals (Hodges & Gill, 2014).

At this level, medical and management staff can also lead processes through multidisciplinary cooperation between teams working in different areas of treatment. To do so requires both organizational and personal leadership (McKimm et al., 2022). The priorities, strategies and objectives of various individuals within the system need to be determined. Contacts need to be developed within the system to provide better medical service and lead intraorganizational change at both the clinical and managerial levels (Reich et al., 2016; Yang et al., 2023).

At the micro-personal level, changes in how patients relate to caregivers and others in the system also underscore the personal changes that healthcare professionals and management staff must undergo. For example, leadership is essential in internal and personal processes and in developing emotional and social intelligence. Practice, guiding and mentoring are needed to foster this type of behavior among others, with emphasis on setting a personal example and creating trust and motivation (McKimm et al., 2022; Uhl-Bien & Carsten, 2018; Yang et al., 2023).

For this reason, in recent years the importance of a new type of medical leader has been increasingly acknowledged. Such a leader exemplifies the balance between accountability and autonomy by placing emphasis on teamwork to increase and improve service and treatment results for patients (Oates, 2012). These changes have led to a reassessment of traditional managerial jobs among medical personnel and have blurred the boundaries between doctors and managers. Consequently, clinical leaders have begun to replace traditional doctor-managers (Kuhlmann & Knorring, 2014), leading to the development of the concept of clinical leadership (Larson & Sahlsten, 2016). Yet despite recent efforts in the professional literature to define and map this concept, it remains vague and lacks connotation (Chávez & Yoder, 2015; Fletcher et al., 2023; Guibert-Lacasa & Vázquez-Calatayud, 2022; Mianda & Voce, 2017; Stanley & Stanley, 2018; Whelehan et al., 2021).

The call for developing leadership capabilities at both the clinical and managerial levels has become more and more extensive as the need for changes at all levels of the system becomes evident. Indeed, healthcare leaders must be capable of leading changes not just among people designated for management or those who hold autonomous management jobs but rather at all levels and among all healthcare system workers (McKimm et al., 2022; Swanwick & McKimm, 2017).

These accelerated changes within healthcare organizations call further attention to the need to redefine leadership. The Fourth Revolution (Schwab, 2017) and the disruptive and innovative processes of digital transformation (Christensen, 2013) were further intensified with the outbreak of the COVID-19 pandemic. Starting in December 2020, healthcare systems were forced to cope with accelerated changes within an extremely short period of time and to implement extensive changes in their business, service and treatment processes (Argenziano et al., 2020).

These processes offered an immediate solution for a system attempting to cope with a health crisis that required providing a response to an unknown, high-risk, and extremely contagious illness, despite a shortage of manpower and resources, increased burnout, and economic instability. These rapid adaptations fundamentally disrupted traditional healthcare practices, leading to the accelerated adoption of telemedicine, restructured care delivery models, and innovative resource management strategies. As a result, the continued implementation of these processes still constitutes a managerial and leadership challenge, demanding ongoing adjustments and resilience from healthcare organizations (Argenziano et al., 2020; Naamati-Schneider & Zaks, 2021; Naamati-Schneider et al., 2024a, 2024b; Zangrandi et al., 2020).

Promoting Clinical Leadership

The concept of leadership and its place in the world of medicine and medical management are still vague. Nevertheless, there is a consensus regarding the importance of leadership capabilities in healthcare organizations and among healthcare workers and patients. For example, promoting clinical leadership among nurses was found to exert a direct influence on treatment outcomes, on the experiences of both caregivers and patients, on staff performance and on treatment quality and safety (Chappell & Richards, 2015; O'Donovan et al., 2021).

Shanafelt et al. (2015) also found that the implementation of effective clinical leadership among doctors was positively associated with decreased staff burnout and fewer medical errors. Yet despite the overwhelming consensus among researchers and healthcare professionals, a large gap still remains between assimilating these processes among management and healthcare professionals and measuring their effectiveness in healthcare organizations (Guibert-Lacasa & Vázquez-Calatayud, 2022). Upon examining the assimilation of leadership capabilities and business acumen among nursing leaders, Raftery et al. (2022) found that development and training in business leadership among nurses is still limited. The researchers emphasized the importance of leadership training as well as the potential offered by business leadership abilities among healthcare managers and professionals.

These and other studies reveal the strong necessity for assimilating planned and managed adaptation processes within healthcare systems and organizations, underscoring the need to adopt transformative leadership models. Various solutions and modes of action are clearly needed to strengthen healthcare system management and establish the need for professional leadership. Building and developing these abilities within healthcare professions will ensure a more secure future for healthcare organizations (Briggs & Isouard, 2016). The global understanding that clinical and managerial medical leadership is important and the perception that leadership is not an inborn trait but can be developed and controlled have led to the development of various training frameworks. These tools and programs are not necessarily a general recipe for personal or organizational success. Nevertheless, they can serve as a "lexicon" that healthcare organizations and individuals can use to discuss the nature of leadership and the ideological relations within their organizations (Swanwick & McKimm, 2017).

Leadership Training Programs

A review of the literature on leadership development reveals many significant differences between traditional and non-traditional leadership training. According to Berkovich and Eyal (2020), traditional training entails the development of managerial skills whereas non-traditional training, which is becoming more widely accepted, involves developing and acquiring action-directed skills that also depend upon the values and identity of each individual. Non-traditional training is expanding and is empowering circumstantial learning, which involves knowledge and skills taken from practical fieldwork, case studies, simulations and more. We now review several of these programs and their implementations in the fields of medicine and medical management.

Management and Leadership Programs and Tools for Enhancing and Assessing Healthcare Leadership Competencies

The change processes described in this book present significant challenges for managers and leaders working in the field of healthcare. Without training or direction in healthcare management, the difficulties facing the system and its workers will become more severe. Indeed, healthcare management is essential at all levels of the healthcare system (Bitkina et al., 2020; Wang & Preininger, 2019). Consequently, in recent decades management training in medical management and leadership has become the topic of intensified research to meet the changing needs of the system and the changing local and global environmental conditions (Counte et al., 2019; Global Consortium for Healthcare Management Professionalization, 2015; Hahn & Lapetra, 2019).

In this context, leadership abilities and behaviors must be developed that include task communication and management, establishing priorities, assimilating change processes, and practical theories. Other important capabilities include analyzing problems, encouraging thought processes and decision-making, and creating a multicultural organizational culture that can foster mutual trust, instill a sense of mission, and enable the development of a common organizational vision and objective. Together these capabilities will enable organizations to adopt change and will encourage innovation, creativity, and variety.

The above steps are essential for grounding the system and preparing it to survive in the present and the future (Global Consortium for Healthcare Management Professionalization, 2015). For example, leadership development programs in the health professions, nursing and occupational therapy have been converted to encompass various objectives and operative tasks, forming the curriculum of a reflection-based pilot program at the Virginia Commonwealth University (VCU) for achieving proactive leadership (Copolillo et al., 2010).

Kouzes and Posner (2013, 2016) also investigated leadership as a collection of skills that can be developed, among them setting a personal example, inspiring a vision, asking questions while attaining objectives, operating outside one's comfort zone, and encouraging creativity, and including the ability to assess the success of all those working within the system. Kouzes and Posner (2013) proposed the Leadership Practices Inventory (LPI) for examining self-leadership and assessing the leadership of others. The LPI is a tool designed to assess an individual's leadership competencies and provide guidance in applying the five practices of the exemplary leadership model to practical organizational challenges. These practices include (1) modeling the way; (2) inspiring a shared vision; (3) challenging the process; (4) enabling others to act; and (5) encouraging the heart. (e.g., demonstrating personal responsibility, challenging the status quo by embracing change and taking calculated risks, empowering team members by encouraging collaboration, building trust, and enabling others to act, and demonstrating empathy by showing genuine care and concern for the well-being of team members). Additionally, the Leadership Development Planner offers a range of developmental activities for leaders to enhance their leadership skills. By understanding how individuals learn to lead and integrating the best leadership learning practices into their routines, leaders can use this tool to further their leadership development.

Similarly, in 2022 the American College of Healthcare Executives published the Healthcare Executive Competency Assessment Tool (ACHE) for examining leadership and management skills among executives and leaders in healthcare systems and organizations across the globe (American College of Healthcare Executives, 2022). The ACHE is grounded in job analysis surveys of healthcare leaders across various management and administration disciplines, ensuring that the competencies are aligned with the challenges and opportunities experienced by today's leaders.

The ACHE competencies are categorized into five domains: communication and relationship management; leadership; professionalism; knowledge of the healthcare environment; and business skills and knowledge. Each domain is defined in detail, and the skills and behaviors necessary for effective healthcare leadership are outlined. Among the competencies are establishing and maintaining relationships, inspiring organizational excellence, aligning personal and organizational conduct with ethical and professional standards, understanding the healthcare system and the environment in which healthcare managers and providers function, and applying business principles to the healthcare environment.

The ACHE can be used at the personal micro level for identifying strengths and weaknesses from the perspective of ACHE competencies. It can also be used to identify common goals, leadership abilities and team cooperation among work teams. At the meso-level this tool can be used to identify performance and organizational processes. At the system-wide macro level it can help identify how processes such as education and development of leadership abilities are planned and assimilated in organizations and individuals. Yet the use of these tools at the system–wide, organizational and personal levels is still insufficient (Hahn & Lapetra, 2019).

Otter (2019) reviewed the development and application of transformative leadership policies in healthcare organizations as part of their adaptation to the changing world. He noted that successful adaptation does not only entail structural reorganization or augmenting the personal abilities and performance of medical professionals. He also claimed that for leaders and managers to lead complex organizations via dynamic processes they must adopt a different way of viewing organizations and leadership. They must also lead organizational action plans for developing value-based leadership. Otter's article describes a case study: a program for developing leadership that was assimilated in a medical center in Norway over a two-year period.

The program focused on identifying personal and team values as the main method for improving leadership abilities among individuals in the organization. This case study demonstrated the difficulties and challenges posed by the need to adapt to the ever-changing, uncertain, complex and vague conditions in which healthcare organizations are forced to function. Yet despite initial opposition, the case study underscored the importance of fostering conditions for leadership as a key to effectiveness. This is especially true in transformative leadership situations that can bridge gaps and serve as the missing link between management and medical treatment. For example, such a leader can act as a mediator between managers and doctors, consequently serving as a crucial link that enhances collaboration and understanding.

Guibert-Lacasa and Vázquez-Calatayud (2022) mapped intervention programs designed to develop interpersonal and personal cognitive leadership abilities among hospital nurses. These programs, implemented over the last decade, included practical problem-solving, making good decisions and controlling learning and behavior (Shen et al., 2018), discussion groups and role-play activities (Chappell & Richards, 2015; Shen et al., 2018), and communications and social skills through mentoring (Leggat et al., 2016).

Programs designed to foster abilities to empower the individual are also being developed and implemented. These programs facilitate development and accepting responsibility, decision-making and self-control, as well as a variety of abilities in the area of emotional intelligence. The programs make use of case studies and professional dilemmas (Leggat et al., 2016). For example, MacPhee et al. (2014) described the development of reflective abilities and self-awareness through use of individual mentoring.

A review by Guibert-Lacasa and Vazquez-Calatayud (2022) reveals the increasing need for a supportive and comprehensive organizational environment to enable healthcare personnel to adopt programs and methodologies such as simulation, role-playing games and case studies. The researchers discuss the limitations of intervention programs while evaluating their effectiveness in developing abilities and their repercussions upon patients. Due to significant differences in the definition of terms and the changing need for various abilities, there is no uniformity in assimilating or assessing these processes, making it difficult to obtain clear-cut results. Consequently, researchers are calling for additional studies and the development of programs and assessment indexes (Guibert-Lacasa & Vázquez-Calatayud, 2022).

Lisevick et al. (2023) described a novel medical student leadership development curriculum that incorporates core elements of lifestyle medicine and emotional intelligence, reflecting a relationship-centered leadership model. The model comprises three leadership domains that are built sequentially and provide a sound basis for longitudinal leadership development as medical training progresses from undergraduate studies to residency and practice.

Discussion

These aforementioned examples demonstrate the changes in perception in healthcare systems and organizations over the past few decades regarding the growing need for developing leadership capabilities among management and healthcare professionals. Nevertheless, there has been no corresponding development of comprehensive leadership capabilities at all levels of management as part of this perceptual change and the need to adopt transformative leadership.

Hence, more and more programs are being offered for developing leadership model skills, such as personal development, teamwork, team management, team building, service delivery, care processes, and the care environment needed to ensure delivery of high quality and safe services. These programs form an integral part of the perception that leadership abilities in the healthcare system must be enhanced. Nevertheless, many differences still remain between the content of these programs and the ability to assess their effectiveness. Moreover, various countries worldwide and even organizations in the same country or region implement these programs differently (Hengy et al., 2023; Matsas et al., 2022; Mianda & Voce, 2017; Sadowski et al., 2018).

It is important to remember that leadership takes place on all levels: personal, interpersonal, organizational and system. Hence, leaders must be familiar with and able to navigate these levels. Assimilation and implementation of leadership capabilities at all levels will make the healthcare system more sustainable and able to adapt to changes, thus facilitating greater stability within an ever-changing, turbulent market.

Indeed, to create strong leadership management the healthcare system must adopt and assimilate these development processes. Moreover, the system must understand the processes of change in the market and their repercussions for all levels of the system (Greenwald, 2017; Lisevick et al., 2023). Leaders and managers in the healthcare system must be capable of quickly assessing these changes and their repercussions. They must then adapt themselves and their organization and lead it toward change while creating appropriate programs for assimilating change (Ginter et al., 2018). Exclusive dependence upon clinical training without emphasizing medical management while developing soft skills and leadership capabilities will slow down processes of innovation and change, causing long-term damage to the stability and strength of the healthcare system (Srinivasan & Chandwani, 2014).

Most studies today focus primarily on intervention programs that take place at later stages of professional training in organizations and less on those that occur during the early stages. They focus on work-based learning methods (WBL) that are implemented within the healthcare organization environment and emphasize personal development. (Guibert-Lacasa & Vázquez-Calatayud, 2022; Mianda & Voce, 2017). Yet we must understand that this process is not personal but rather organizational. It is not a one-time occurrence but rather a long-term process that must be implemented at all levels of the organization throughout all stages of training. Hence the extent of these programs should be expanded to encompass early training up to advanced professional in-service-training. Other players should also be involved, such as institutions of higher education and medical education as well as healthcare organizations (McKimm et al., 2022).

Moreover, emphasis should be placed on a general holistic leadership process that includes the development of such necessary capabilities as cognitive skills, soft personal and interpersonal abilities based on comprehensive learning methods such as work-based learning (WBL), personal practice and mentoring, and team learning while developing lifelong learning capabilities (Mianda & Voce, 2017). Developing leadership in the healthcare system should also focus on education in all realms of management and treatment to transform workers at all levels into proactive workers capable of inspiring, motivating, training and mentoring others in these adaptation processes (McKimm et al., 2022).

In a world marked by accelerated change and the increased use of shared processes, holacratic leadership may be the most appropriate form of leadership for service organizations such as health organizations and services (Mazilu & Dobrescu, 2020). A combination of adaptive management, holacratic management and treatment teams should create leadership models that are specific to the healthcare system and suit the market and the environment. This will necessitate long-term planning and comprehensive allotment of resources for developing and assimilating cognitive, interpersonal and personal leadership capabilities.

Early planning and understanding expected difficulties while determining criteria and establishing uniform definitions, goals and measurement methods will make it possible to train professional manpower in a timely manner while planning changes holistically. Doing so will contribute to system stability and sustainability and in turn enable healthcare systems to provide improved services for everyone (Figueroa et al., 2019).

References

Ahlsson, A. (2020) Why change? Lessons in leadership from the COVID-19 pandemic. *European Journal of Cardiothorac Surgery* 1, *58*(3), 411–413. https://doi.org/10.1093/ejcts/ezaa252

American College of Healthcare Executives. (2022). *ACHE healthcare executive competencies assessment tool*. Retrieved from https://www.ache.org/-/media/ache/career-resource-center/cat-2022.pdf

Anthony, W. A., & Huckshorn, K. A. (2008). *Principled leadership in mental health systems and programs*. Boston University.

Argenziano, M., Fischkoff, K., & Smith, C. R. (2020). Surgery scheduling in a crisis. *New England Journal of Medicine*. https://doi.org/10.1056/NEJMc2017424

Berkovich, I., & Eyal, O. (2020). Ethics education in leadership development: Adopting multiple ethical paradigms. *Educational Management Administration and Leadership, 48*(2), 270–285. https://doi.org/10.1177/1741143218792914

Bernstein, E., Bunch, J., Canner, N., & Lee, M. (2016). Beyond the holacracy hype. In *Harvard Business Review*, (July-August) (pp. 2–13). https://hbr.org/2016/07/beyond-the-holacracy-hype

Bitkina, O. V., Kim, H. K., & Park, J. (2020). Usability and user experience of medical devices: An overview of the current state, analysis methodologies, and future challenges. *International Journal of Industrial Ergonomics, 76*, 102932. https://doi.org/10.1016/j.ergon.2020.102932

Briggs, D., & Isouard, G. (2016). The language of health reform and health management: critical issues in the management of health systems. *Asia Pacific Journal of Health Management, 11*(3), 38–44. https://doi.org/10.24083/apjhm.v11i3.153

Bruce, J., McKee, K., Morgan-Fleming, J., & Warner, W. (2019). The Oaks leadership scholars program: Transformative leadership in action. *International Journal of Teaching and Learning in Higher Education, 31*(3), 536–546.

Burns, J. M. (2012). *Leadership.* Open Road Media.

Cernega, A., Nicolescu, D. N., Meleşcanu Imre, M., Ripszky Totan, A., Arsene, A. L., Şerban, R. S., Perpelea, A. C., Nedea, M. I., & Piţuru, S. M. (2024). Volatility, uncertainty, complexity, and ambiguity (VUCA) n healthcare. *Healthcare, 12*(7), 773. https://doi.org/10.3390/healthcare12070773

Chappell, K. B., & Richards, K. C. (2015). New graduate nurses, new graduate nurse transition programs, and clinical leadership skill. *Journal for Nurses in Professional Development, 31*(3), 128-E8. https://doi.org/10.1097/NND.0000000000000159

Chávez, E. C., & Yoder, L. H. (2015). Staff nurse clinical leadership: A concept analysis. *Nursing Forum, 50*(2), 90–100. https://doi.org/10.1111/nuf.12100

Choflet, A., Packard, T., & Stashower, K. (2021). Rethinking organizational change in the COVID-19 era. *Journal of Hospital Management and Health Policy, 5*, 16.

Christensen, C. M. (2013). *The innovator's dilemma: When new technologies cause great firms to fail.* Harvard Business Review Press.

Copolillo, A., Shepherd, J., Anzalone, M., & Lane, S. J. (2010). Taking on the challenge of the centennial vision: Transforming the passion for occupational therapy into a passion for leadership. *Occupational Therapy in Health Care, 24*(1), 7–22. https://doi-org.mgs.hac.ac.il/10.3109/07380570903304209

Counte, M. A., Howard, S. W., Chang, L., & Aaronson, W. (2019). Global advances in value-based payment and their implications for global health management education, development, and practice. *Frontiers in Public Health, 6*, 379. https://doi.org/10.3389/fpubh.2018.00379

Ewens, A. (2002). The nature and purpose of leadership. In E. Hawkins & C. Thornton (Eds.), *Managing and leading innovation in health care.* Harcour.

Figueroa, C. A., Harrison, R., Chauhan, A., & Meyer, L. (2019). Priorities and challenges for health leadership and workforce management globally: A rapid review. *BMC Health Services Research, 19*(1), 1–11. https://doi.org/10.1186/s12913-019-4080-7

Fletcher, M., Read, C., D-Adderio, L. (2023). Nurse leadership post COVID pandemic—a framework for digital healthcare innovation and transformation. *SAGE Open Nursing, 9*. https://doi.org/10.1177/23779608231160465

Ginter, P. M., Duncan, W. J., & Swayne, L. E. (2018). *The strategic management of health care organizations.* John Wiley & Sons.

Global Consortium for Healthcare Management Professionalization. (2015). *Leadership Competencies for Healthcare Services Managers.* International Hospital Federation. Available online at: https://www.ihf-fih.org/download_doc_file.php?doc=dfff684f5fd4854ad43566085950b8a8

Goleman, D. (2017). Leadership that gets results. In *Leadership perspectives* (pp. 85–96). Routledge.

Greenwald, H. P. (2017). Management challenges in British Columbia's healthcare system. *Journal of Health Organization and Management, 31*(4), 418–429. https://doi.org/10.1108/JHOM-03-2017-0059

Guibert-Lacasa, C., & Vázquez-Calatayud, M. (2022). Nurses, clinical leadership in the hospital setting: A systematic review. *Journal of Nursing Management, 30*(4), 913–925. https://doi.org.mgs.hac.ac.il/10.1111/jonm.13570

Hahn, C. A., & Gil Lapetra, M. (2019). Development and use of the leadership competencies for healthcare services managers assessment. *Frontiers in Public Health, 7*, 34. https://doi.org/10.3389/fpubh.2019.00034

Heifetz, R. A., Heifetz, R., Grashow, A., & Linsky, M. (2009). *The practice of adaptive leadership: Tools and tactics for changing your organization and the world*. Harvard business press.

Hengy, M., Farooqui, S., Dimitrion, P., Fotouhi, A., & Daveluy, S. (2023). Leadership training in dermatology: A narrative review. *International Journal of Dermatology, 62*(1), 97–102. https://doi-org.mgs.hac.ac.il/10.1111/ijd.16510

Hodges, J., & Gill, R. (2014). *Sustaining change in organizations*. Sage.

House, R. J. (1971). A path goal theory of leader effectiveness. *Administrative Science Quarterly*, 321–339.

Kotter, J. P. (2008). *Force for change: How leadership differs from management*. Simon and Schuster.

Kouzes, J. M., & Posner, B. Z. (2013). *Leadership practices inventory* (4th ed.). Pefeiffer.

Kouzes, J. M., & Posner, B. Z. (2016). *The leadership challenge: How to make extraordinary things happen in organizations* (6th ed.). John Wiley & Sons Inc.

Kuhlmann, E., & von Knorring, M. (2014). Management and medicine: Why we need a new approach to the relationship. *Journal of Health Services Research and Policy, 19*, 189–191. https://doi.org/10.1177/1355819614524946

Larsson, I. E., & Sahlsten, M. J. (2016). The staff nurse clinical leader at the Bedside: Swedish registered nurses' perceptions. *Nursing Research and Practice, 1*, 1797014. https://doi.org/10.1155/2016/1797014

Laverack, G. (2014). *The pocket guide to health promotion*. McGraw-Hill Education (UK).

Leggat, S. G., Smyth, A., Balding, C., & McAlpine, I. (2016). Equipping clinical leaders for system and service improvements in quality and safety: An Australian experience. *Australian and New Zealand Journal of Public Health, 40*(2), 138–143. https://doi.org/10.1111/1753-6405.12462

Lisevick, A., Dreiling, J., Chauvin, S., Falisi, S., Feinn, R., Gulati, M., Frates, B., & Anand, R. (2023). Leadership for medical students: Lessons learned from a relationship-centered leadership curriculum. *American Journal of Lifestyle Medicine, 17*(1), 56–63. https://doi-org.mgs.hac.ac.il/10.1177/15598276221106940

MacPhee, M. , Dahinten, V. S. , Hejazi, S. , Laschinger, H. , Kazanjian, A. , McCutcheon, A. , Skelton-Green, J. , & O'Brien-Pallas, L. (2014). Testing the effects of an empowerment-based leadership development programme: Part 1—Leader outcomes. *Journal of Nursing Management, 22*(1), 4–15.

Maeda, K., & Socha-Dietrich, K. (2021). Skills for the future health workforce: Preparing health professionals for people-centred care. *OECD Health Working Papers, 124*. https://doi.org/10.1787/68fb5f08-en

Marcus, L. J., Dorn, B. C., Henderson, J., & McNulty, E. (2015). *Meta-leadership: A framework for building leadership effectiveness*. Harvard University.

Matsas, B., Goralnick, E., Bass, M., Barnett, E., Nagle, B., & Sullivan, E. (2022). Leadership development in U.S. undergraduate medical education: A scoping review of curricular content and competency frameworks. *Academic Medicine, 97*(6), 899–908. https://doi.org/10.1097/ACM.0000000000004632

Mazilu, C. E., & Dobrescu, R. (2020). Increasing autonomy in health care management with teal organizations. *International Conference on e-Health and Bioengineering (EHB), 2020*, 1–4. https://doi.org/10.1109/EHB50910.2020.9280172

McKimm, J., & Jones, P. K. (2018). Twelve tips for applying change models to curriculum design, development and delivery. *Medical Teacher, 40*(5), 520–526. https://doi.org/10.1080/0142159X.2017.1391377

Mianda, S., & Voce, A. S. (2017). Conceptualizations of clinical leadership: A review of the literature. *Journal of Healthcare Leadership, 9*, 79–87. https://doi.org/10.2147/JHL.S143639

McKimm, J., Ramani, S., Forrest, K., Bishop, J., Findyartini, A., Mills, C., Hassanien, M., Al-Hayani, A., Jones, P., Nadarajah, V.D., & Radu, G. (2022). Adaptive leadership during challenging times: Effective strategies for health professions educators: AMEE guide No. 148. *Medical Teacher*, 1–11. https://doi.org/10.1080/0142159X.2022.2057288

Naamati-Schneider, L. (2020). Strategic management as adaptation to changes in the ecosystems of public hospitals in Israel. *Israel Journal Health Policy Resources*, *9*, 65. https://doi.org/10.1186/s13584-020-00424-y

Naamati-Schneider, L. (2022). Intraorganization conflicts of interest in hospitals adapting to a changing ecosystem. *Journal of Health Organization and Management, 36*(3), 265–278. https://doi.org/10.1108/JHOM-09-2021-0325

Naamati-Schneider, L. (2023). The effect of digitalization on service orientation and service perception among Israeli healthcare professionals: A qualitative study. *Digital Health, 9*. https://doi.org/10.1177/20552076231191892

Naamati-Schneider, L., & Salvatore, F. P. (2023). Sustainability for healthcare organisations and systems: Cultivating strategy and governance processes for a better future. In D. Vrontis, A. Thrassou, L. Efthymiou, Y. Weber, S. M. R. Shams, & E. Tsoukatos, (Eds.), *Business for sustainability, volume I. Palgrave studies in cross-disciplinary business research, in association with EuroMed Academy of Business*. Palgrave Macmillan. https://doi.org/10.1007/978-3-031-37361-9_11

Naamati-Schneider, L., & Zaks, O. (2021). Public hospitals in crisis: Managerial and strategic adaptation. In D. Vrontis, A. Thrassou, Y. Weber, S. M. R. Shams, E. Tsoukatos, & L. Efthymiou (Eds.), *Business under crisis, Volume II. Palgrave studies in cross-disciplinary business research, in association with EuroMed Academy of Business*. Palgrave Macmillan, Cham. https://doi.org/10.1007/978-3-030-76575-0_3

Naamati-Schneider, L., Arazi-Fadlon, M., & Daphna-Tekoah, S. (2024a). Strategic technological processes in hospitals: Conflicts and personal experiences of healthcare teams. *Nursing Ethics*. https://doi.org/10.1177/09697330241252876

Naamati-Schneider, L., Arazi-Fadlon, M., & Daphna-Tekoah, S. (2024b). Navigating moral and ethical dilemmas and conflict in strategic technological processes within healthcare organizations. *Digital Health*.

Nelson, T., & Squires, V. (2017). Addressing complex challenges through adaptive leadership: A promising approach to collaborative problem solving. *Journal of Leadership Education, 16*(4). https://doi.org/10.12806/V16/I4/T2

Northouse, P. (2011). Leadership: Theory and practice (6th ed). Sage.

O'Donovan, R., Rogers, L., Khurshid, Z., De Brún, A., Nicholson, E., O'Shea, M., Ward, M., & McAuliffe, E. (2021). A systematic review exploring the impact of focal leader behaviours on health care team performance. *Journal of Nursing Management, 29*(6), 1420–1443. https://doi.org/10.1111/jonm.13403

Oates, K. (2012). The new clinical leader. *Journal of Paediatrics and Child Health, 48*(6), 472–475. https://doi.org/10.1111/j.1440-1754.2012.02478.x

Otter, K. (2019). Developing leadership: innovation, adaptability and integration in large-scale health care organizations. *Experten führen: Modelle, Ideen und Praktiken für die Organisations- und Führungsentwicklung*, 179–192. https://doi.org/10.1007/978-3-658-23028-9_10

Raftery, C., Sassenberg, A. M., & Bamford-Wade, A. (2022). Business acumen for nursing leaders: An exploratory qualitative study. *Journal of Nursing Management*. https://doi.org/10.1111/jonm.13672

Reich, M. R., Javadi, D., & Ghaffar, A. (2016). Introduction to the special issue on effective leadership for health systems. *Health Systems and Reform, 2*(3), 171–175. https://doi.org/10.1080/23288604.2016.1223978

Robertson, B. J. (2007) Organization at the leading edge: Introducing holacracy™, *Integral Leadership Review, 7*(3).

Sadowski, B., Cantrell, S., Barelski, A., O'Malley, P. G., & Hartzell, J. D. (2018). Leadership training in graduate medical education: A systematic review. *Journal of Graduate Medical Education, 10*, 134–148.

Schwab, K. (2017). *The fourth industrial revolution*. Currency.

Senkubuge, F., Modisenyane, M., & Bishaw, T. (2014). Strengthening health systems by health sector reforms. *Global Health Action, 7*(1), 23568. https://doi.org/10.3402/gha.v7.23568
Shanafelt, T. D., Gorringe, G., Menaker, R., Storz, K. A., Reeves, D., Buskirk, S. J., et al. (2015). Impact of organizational leadership on physician burnout and satisfaction. *Mayo Clinic Proceedings, 90*, 432–440. https://doi.org/10.1016/j.mayocp.2015.01.012
Shen, Q., Peltzer, J., Teel, C., & Pierce, J. (2018). Kansas nurse leader residency programme: Advancing leader knowledge and skills. *Journal of Nursing Management, 26*(2), 148–157. https://doi.org/10.1111/jonm.12527
Srinivasan, V., & Chandwani, R. (2014). HRM innovations in rapid growth contexts: The healthcare sector in India. *The International Journal of Human Resource Management, 25*(10), 1505–1525. https://doi.org/10.1080/09585192.2013.870308
Stanley, D., & Stanley, K. (2018). Clinical leadership and nursing explored: A literature search. *Journal of Clinical Nursing, 27*(9–10), 1730–1743. https://doi.org/10.1111/jocn.14145
Swanwick, T., & McKimm, J. (2017). *ABC of clinical leadership*. John Wiley & Sons.
Uhl-Bien, M., & Carsten, M. (2018). Reversing the lens in leadership: Positioning followership in the leadership construct. *Leadership now: Reflections on the legacy of Boas Shamir* (pp. 195–225). Bingley.
van Diggele, C., Burgess, A., Roberts, C., & Mellis, C. (2020). Leadership in healthcare education. *BMC Medical Education, 20*(2), 1–6. https://doi.org/10.1186/s12909-020-02288-x
Wang, F., & Preininger, A. (2019). AI in health: State of the art, challenges, and future directions. *Yearbook of Medical Informatics, 28*(01), 016–026.
Whelehan, D. F., Algeo, N., & Brown, D. A. (2021). Leadership through crisis: Fighting the fatigue pandemic in healthcare during COVID-19. *BMJ Leader, 5*(2), 108–112. https://doi.org/10.1136/leader-2020-000419
World Health Organization. (2016). Global diffusion of eHealth: Making universal health coverage achievable. World Health Organisation. Retrieved November 10, 2022, from http://apps.who.int/iris/bitstream/10665/252529/1/9789241511780-eng.pdf?ua=1
World Health Organization. (2019). Universal health coverage. Retrieved from https://www.who.int/news-room/fact-sheets/detail/universal-health-coverage-(uhc)
Worley, C. G., & Jules, C. (2020). COVID-19's uncomfortable revelations about agile and sustainable organizations in a VUCA world. *The Journal of Applied Behavioral Science, 56*(3), 279–283. https://doi.org/10.1177/0021886320936263
Yang, P., Diaz, A., Chhabra, K. R., Byrnes, M. E., Rajkumar, A., Nathan, H., & Dimick, J. B. (2023). Surgical leadership competencies for navigating hospital network expansion. *Journal of Surgical Research, 283*, 76–83. https://doi.org/10.1016/j.jss.2022.10.014
Zangrandi, A., Fanelli, S., Donelli, C. C., & Elefanti, M. (2020). *Crisis managment: la gestione di un ospedale durante una pandemia*. EGEA.

Chapter 10
Customer/Patient Service Orientation: Nurturing Service Competencies in Healthcare Systems

Abstract Adapting to environmental changes in healthcare requires a well-trained workforce with a strong service orientation and the necessary competencies. This chapter delves into the transformations in customer service orientation and patient-centered care within the healthcare system at macro, meso, and micro levels. It outlines essential educational practices for training healthcare professionals at both managerial and clinical levels to adapt to these changes. By describing methodological tools and intervention plans for students and staff, the chapter aims to ensure the continuity of high-quality care and enhance the efficiency and stability of the healthcare system over the long term.

Introduction

Healthcare systems across the globe must face numerous challenges brought on by changing environments and dynamic and uncertain conditions. To meet evolving healthcare demands and still remain competitive, healthcare organizations have been forced to change and adapt to cope with global and local shifts, including rising costs and quality concerns (Denis & van Gestel, 2015; Naamati-Schneider, 2020, 2021). These changes are reflected at all levels of the healthcare system: the macro level (e.g., government bodies and international organizations that formulate policies; regulations and funding mechanisms that set the agenda for healthcare delivery); the meso level (e.g., hospitals, HMOs, clinics and community health centers that are responsible for managing and delivering health services); and the micro levels (e.g., direct interaction between caregivers and patients, medical treatment, counselling). Each of these levels plays a crucial role in delivering healthcare services to the population.

Healthcare systems have begun adopting a competitive business agenda as part of their attempt to adapt to a competitive market while maintaining an economic balance. In addition, the quantity and variety of the services they provide is constantly increasing, necessitating a broader emphasis and a more holistic view of patients'

L. Naamati-Schneider and D. Alt, *Technology and Competency-Oriented Learning*,
https://doi.org/10.1007/978-981-97-5771-8_10

physical, mental and social well-being (Erkan & Unal, 2022; Maeda & Socha-Dietrich, 2021; Naamati-Schneider & Salvatore, 2023; Sriatmi et al., 2020). The issue of service has consequently become an important and dominant component, and resources are being devoted to the central position patients have begun to assume in healthcare services and treatment. Indeed, the conduct of healthcare systems worldwide reflects the importance attributed to this issue (Henrike & Schultz, 2014).

By adopting patient-oriented processes, an organization can differentiate itself, establish its reputation and achieve a high standing in the competitive market. Consequently, if an organization and its workers wish to survive and adapt to the changing market, such strategies must be adopted by its management, within its organizational culture and among its managers and professionals (Singh, 2012).

The transition from the patronizing approach that previously characterized healthcare services, an approach that emphasized the needs of the caregivers, marks a significant change in perception in healthcare systems (Richards et al., 2013). This shift is also reflected in a change in administered treatment methods, which in the past concentrated only on clinical outcomes as an index. This patronizing approach has been replaced by an approach that places the customer/patient at the center. This new approach incorporates many other service-oriented features, such as accessibility, availability, ongoing treatment, continuity and attitude toward patients. It also encompasses organizational service-oriented aspects, such as proper use of resources, avoiding duplication, and organizational quality (Aka Zohar, 2019).

As such, the healthcare system and the professionals within it are currently transitioning towards patient-centered care (Jarva et al., 2023; Maeda & Socha-Dietrich, 2021). This transition required extensive changes at all levels, including a shift to patient-caregiver relationships that foster equality, cooperation and patient empowerment. These changes occurred simultaneously with growing awareness of patient consumerism and access to information, changes in the balance of power in patient-caregiver relationships, and changes in patients' expectations from their healthcare system. Indeed, today patients assess healthcare organizations no differently than they assess other business organizations that provide them services. This attitude challenges the healthcare system to meet the needs of their customers—the patients.

The outbreak of the COVID-19 pandemic at the end of 2019 generated numerous and far-reaching changes related to digital technology assimilation that resulted in changes in how healthcare organizations provided services. These changes are expected to be assimilated into the system and create a new reality. For example, information has become accessible for both caregivers and patients, necessitating significant organizational and personnel changes across the entire system to accommodate the new working methods. Among these changes are long-distance medicine, the use of robotics and new medical instrumentation and technology, and online services (Kraus et al., 2021; Marques & Ferreira, 2020; Naamati-Schneider & Zaks, 2022). These changes have far-reaching repercussions for medical staff members and healthcare organizations, which must assimilate and adapt to patient-centered care and the services to support it (Aka Zohar, 2019; Birk, 2019; Naamati-Schneider, 2022, 2023) while at the same time striving to increase the system's long-range efficiency and quality.

This chapter reviews the ramifications of the environmental changes necessitated by a service orientation on the three levels noted above—macro, meso and micro—each of which plays a crucial role in the delivery of health services to the population. The chapter also discusses how this service orientation can be inculcated and what competencies are required for developing it within health organizations, the health system and the managerial and professional staff on each of the three levels. The chapter sheds light on changes in customer service orientation and patient orientation within the health system and outlines the educational practices needed to train the managerial and clinical workforce.

Providing methodological tools and offering intervention programs to students and healthcare professionals in medical management will help clarify the principles of the approach and will create a strong basis for directing and inculcating change. In this way, it will be possible to maintain and sustain the quality of care and service while enabling the system to provide high-quality service and remain more efficient and stable over time.

Customer/Patient Service Orientation

By definition, a service orientation refers to the inclination on the part of service providers to be helpful, thoughtful, considerate and cooperative. Such an inclination encompasses a range of attitudes and behaviors that influence the nature and quality of the interaction between an organization's staff and its customers, including hospital employees and patients (Hogan et al., 1984).

A service orientation is an essential component of emotional intelligence and constitutes a practical component in hiring and training workers in organizations (Gong et al., 2019; Serrat, 2017). Workers with a high service orientation have good capabilities for interacting with others. Consequently they can serve as trustworthy emissaries of the organization when meeting with clients and can meet clients' needs and expectations. In the field of healthcare, service can be defined as an intangible benefit that cannot be physically viewed, felt, counted, touched or measured like other manufactured goods.

Service is an inseparable part of an organization's chain of values. It also plays a significant and dominant role in building and assimilating a competitive strategy. Hence, service encompasses values and resources and offers an opportunity to differentiate companies and promote their relative advantages (Porter & Lee, 2016). The quality of healthcare service depends upon the patients/customers, the service providers and the interaction between them. For this reason, service is not always homogeneous or well-defined, even within a specific organization (Endeshaw, 2021; Lagrosen & Lagrosen, 2022; Vaish et al., 2016; Yang & Yoon, 2023). A service orientation implies determining a direction for the various services and products that an organization provides to benefit its clients/patients (Tung et al., 2014). In the context of the processes of change now characterizing healthcare systems and organizations, patients are becoming more and more active players. They exert more control over decision-making and are more exposed to various alternatives. The growing reliance on service orientation processes has generated customer-centered organizations that offer professional services while creating a competitive advantage and improving performance and results that benefit customers (Gilbert & Laporte, 2023; Vaish et al., 2016).

Today, service orientation also falls within the general definition of quality. Organizations must be able to provide service that satisfactorily meets their clients' expectations. For clients, quality service is among the best options available on the market (Ampaw et al., 2020). Service orientation and service direction also entail the establishment of indexes to measure the quality of clinical and service factors. Indeed, organizations can use service processes to deal with competition by creating a competitive advantage in the market (Chang et al., 2013). These change processes are mediated at various levels of the organization, are influenced by organizational climate and ethics, and have repercussions on workers' performance (Halvorsen et al., 2023). An organization's service orientation finds expression at all levels: the macro-system level, the meso-organizational level, and the personal micro level (Naamati-Schneider, 2023).

Service Orientation Manifested on the Macro, Meso and Micro Levels

The Macro Level

Service orientation at the macro level reflects the entire healthcare system and its need to adapt to a changing market that is growing more competitive every day by adopting a broad strategic view (Maeda & Socha-Dietrich, 2021). Changes at this level include the need to regulate the standardization of quality and to establish system-wide codes and regulations. In recent years these changes have also been influenced by legislation that seeks to safeguard patients' rights, maintain their privacy and self-respect, ensure their right to make decisions, provide medical immunity, and other issues as well.

The repercussions at this level also include standardization and setting guidelines to govern planning, budgeting, purchasing and development, as well as assimilation of new digital technologies that will facilitate efficient, sustainable, high-quality service (Vyas et al., 2023). To further enhance the professionalism of healthcare service providers, educational processes must be planned, budgeted and incorporated, and service skills must be cultivated within the curricula of medical, nursing and other health-related programs. These programs should include training in health system management to ensure that students are well-equipped to meet the evolving needs of the healthcare industry and to facilitate professional development among all service providers in the healthcare system (Dolev et al., 2021; Fenton et al., 2012; Halvorsen et al., 2023).

The Organizational Meso Level

Service orientation finds expression in several ways at the meso level of an organization: in planning and budgeting to develop and assimilate digital technologies that enable client-oriented service, in using technological aids and in adapting the system to online service (Vyas et al., 2023). At the same time, the system must help management and clinical staff become familiar with organizational and cultural change processes at all levels (Gilbert & Laporte, 2023). Staff members must be involved in determining the organization's vision, values and culture in a way that emphasizes cultural capability, while at the same time placing patients and their families at the center. Emphasis must also be placed on developing interpersonal communication skills, making services more accessible, creating a marketing setup suitable to clients, and developing awareness of service orientation among medical and managerial staff. Organizational standards and processes must be developed and assimilated to ensure that patients have a positive experience, among other things by providing appropriate information, empowering patients, guaranteeing safety during treatment, ensuring proper conditions in the physical plant, maintaining treatment continuity and fostering respectful relations (Gilbert & Laporte, 2023).

Other organizational characteristics, among them accessibility, availability and service, have been found to be directly connected to patients' perceptions of the patient-caregiver relationship. For example, lengthy waiting times and short-lived consultations are a direct result of organizational regulations. Visit regulations, schedules and budgets all are liable to have a direct impact on patients' perceptions and the patient-caregiver relationship. Healthcare service organizations that have adopted a customer orientation are becoming increasingly aware of the need for assimilating these changes at the various levels. Tools have been developed for measuring and improving patients' experiences to achieve a competitive advantage in the market. The results of annual surveys conducted to measure patient satisfaction are published for the general public, spurring medical institutions to compete for quality service (Aka Zohar, 2019). Alongside organizational changes, other steps include appointing designated administrators to promote service and train staff members, establishing service centers, developing programs and tools for promoting a service orientation among healthcare professionals, and setting and enforcing standards (Maeda & Socha-Dietrich, 2021).

The Personal Micro Level

At the personal micro level, healthcare professionals and managers must deal with a constantly changing system that has had a significant impact on the patient-caregiver relationship in terms of trust, satisfaction and response to treatment. In the past, patient-caregiver relationships were asymmetrical in that the doctor made decisions and the patient accepted them. In the past few years, however, this relationship has changed: Patients have become more actively involved in their treatment, and the gaps between doctors and patients have decreased (Aka Zohar, 2019), resulting in improved patient responses and health (Präg et al., 2017). Treatment is becoming more personal and adapted to the needs of each individual patient. Care is administered with compassion and sensitivity and is based on positive connections with the patient. This patient-centered focus has been found to have a direct influence on patients' responses and their perceptions of treatment quality (Attree, 2001; Fenton et al., 2012; Halvorsen et al., 2023).

Patient-oriented service is based on values that view all individuals as unique, recognize their right to privacy, independence and choice, preserve their rights as equal members of society, and offer respect and inclusion. Patients are also afforded control in making decisions regarding their health and treatment. This type of orientation will empower patients, thus promoting change and a positive response to treatment (Aka Zohar, 2019; Powers & Bendall, 2004). Beyond the nature of the patient-caregiver relationship, patient empowerment depends upon the patient's personality, culture and socioeconomic status. Efforts to make the system more service-oriented and client/patient-centered must consequently focus on cooperation in decision-making, perspectives when setting goals, interpersonal communication, and information transmission and guidance (Gilbert & Laporte, 2023; Powers & Bendall, 2004).

As a result of the availability of medical information on the internet together with patients' ability to interact with other patients, online communities or local patient organizations, health consumers are able to be active partners in using healthcare services. Most patients who have access to information become experts regarding their illness and expect to play an active role in their treatment. Patient cooperation and involvement benefit both patients and caregivers and exert a positive impact on treatment quality and patient satisfaction—two core objectives of healthcare service organizations (Gilbert & Laporte, 2023).

Service-oriented behavior among healthcare professionals involves thinking and planning ahead, planning patients' needs, cooperation, and working with a comprehensive team to benefit patients. Ongoing cooperation and interaction with patients are also essential. When healthcare professionals assimilate the service orientation at the personal level, patients become actively involved and their sense of cooperation is enhanced. Indeed, patients become empowered and are able to develop and accumulate relevant medical knowledge. High-quality communication with patients and their families generates motivation and commitment to treatment response, thus improving patient recuperation as well (Shaller, 2007).

In summary, integrating service awareness and service orientation at all levels fosters and enhances customers' experiences, in turn affecting customers' overall perceptions of the healthcare system throughout their treatment (Aka Zohar, 2019). These experiences are influenced by their encounters with caregivers, the healthcare system as a whole and the entire organizational climate. The combination of a service orientation and customer-centered care as part of customer orientation has already been implemented in numerous organizations at all levels. The result is improved customer experience, customer empowerment, improved treatment response, higher quality and better clinical results. One strategy for adopting these perceptions is based on the principle that the customers' needs must be considered when building the healthcare system while adopting strategies of co-creation and co-design (Gilbert & Laporte, 2023; Zhang et al., 2015). Adopting the customer orientation approach necessitates involving patients in organizational culture processes, in the formulation of treatment policies and in work processes. Indeed, the findings of the MARQuIS Project, a comprehensive in-depth analysis of 371 hospitals across eight countries, corroborated the occurrence of these trends in the healthcare landscape, providing empirical evidence to support their existence. The findings revealed that a high percentage of hospitals have begun to assimilate service-oriented and patient-centered processes by involving patients in decision-making, thinking and implementation at various levels. Patients were also included in policy-making through Learning from Patients program to improve organizational quality and performance (Groene et al., 2009).

The changes described in this chapter and their consequences for service and service quality create new challenges that must be addressed. Contradictions arise regarding treatment methods, new treatment interfaces such as the use of video and tools for online diagnosis, and mobile (M) health. The nature of treatment and the closeness and intimacy of patient-caregiver relationships are also changing. A wide variety of service providers and digital tools are available, yet patients differ in their access to and understanding of digital tools. These differences must be dealt with and implemented by adopting a holistic view within the organization and system. Accordingly, the role of medical managers is also changing, and the needs of the profession are expanding. Those who are implementing these changes within the organization must be trained while simultaneously developing service skills and patient/customer orientation skills among all managers and workers at all levels of the system (Jarva et al., 2023; Maeda & Socha-Dietrich, 2021).

Service Orientation Implementation in Educational Processes

For changes in service orientation and customer orientation to be assimilated, processes of change and competencies must be embedded within all levels of the system. This section reviews the pedagogical processes necessary to achieve this end.

In recent years, the need to recognize these changes and adopt patient-centered strategies has attained increasing validity, leading groups of experts in the fields of medicine, nursing and other healthcare professions toward uniform efforts to identify core competencies that must be developed among workers. The OECD published a report pointing to the necessity of these core work skills (Maeda & Socha-Dietrich, 2021), with the goal of adopting service orientation processes while focusing on the current and future needs and desires of customers/patients. The workers and the organization must assimilate cultural perceptional change processes while developing specific skills found to be connected to a service orientation. Among these skills are personal and interpersonal communication, the ability to see different viewpoints, teamwork, team decision-making, cultural adaptation and avoiding ethnocentric behavior (Jarva et al., 2023). Despite the growing consensus that these skills are necessary for developing and training workers, opinions differ regarding what programs should be used and how they should be incorporated and evaluated at different stages of training in higher education institutions and within medical organizations. In the following section we describe several projects aimed at fostering these skills.

Promoting Cultural Skills

Cultural competence, considered to be a core skill, has become a central issue in organizations. Attempts at both the meso and personal levels to promote cultural competence aim at providing better customer experiences and satisfaction, with the ultimate goal of obtaining a competitive advantage. Cultural and language gaps between caregivers and patients have been found to be connected to communication problems, patient mistrust and dissatisfaction with treatment. In contrast, a robust level of cultural competence among healthcare providers has had a positive influence on various outcomes, including heightened satisfaction among both caregivers and patients, improved patient adherence to treatment plans, and enhanced communication and information sharing. This association between cultural competence and favorable outcomes has been supported by empirical research and is widely acknowledged in the academic literature (Jongen et al., 2018b; Roe et al., 2012; Truong et al., 2014). Jongen et al. (2018a) reviewed 64 intervention programs that offered cultural competence training in Canada, the United States, Australia and New Zealand during the period 2008 through 2015. Despite the apparent need to teach competencies that enable workers to translate knowledge into practical situations and the need to assess the influence of such intervention programs, most of them sought mainly to develop knowledge, awareness and sensitivity among healthcare workers. The terminology and definitions used to describe the concept of cultural competence varied greatly, as did the objectives of these intervention programs. The reviewed programs were designated for all workers in the examined organizations—not only for medical professionals—indicating that cultural competence intervention programs are generic rather than based on skills or knowledge specific to any particular profession.

Studies in the field of cultural competence found that providing staff members with organizational training through intervention programs positively correlated with the organization's level of cultural competence (Truong et al., 2014). Nevertheless, more comprehensive studies are needed on this topic, as are programs to foster and assimilate these competencies and further research to assess their effectiveness (Jongen et al., 2018a, 2018b).

Nurturing Digital Skills

Digital customer relationship management is another area found to be associated with service and customer orientation. The use of digital tools and modern information technologies facilitates understanding and analysis of patients' needs. This area incorporates methodologies as well as knowledge of computer hardware and software that can assist organizations in interacting with customers. What is needed is a system that incorporates marketing activities for new customers along with activities for retaining current customers while assessing the resulting value generated for the organization. Such a system should determine objectives and patient needs, manage patient time, shift workers' focus to a customer orientation, change bureaucratic work methods, set an agenda and clear-cut objectives for a customer orientation, and set and measure quality standards (Kraus et al, 2021; Patricio et al, 2020).

Courses focusing on patient care, quality and safety are becoming increasingly popular in medical schools and medical management programs, and such courses have been required by the OECD since 2012. Health organizations are encouraged to develop programs for assimilating an organizational culture of quality as part of their service. Nevertheless, most indexes for measuring quality focus on clinical quality rather than quality of service (Dreiher et al., 2020). A group of researchers in Finland (Jarva et al., 2023) recently proposed tools for examining digital competence, claiming that these tools can be used to examine intervention programs as well as levels of digital competence among healthcare workers. Their study provided a partial solution to the growing need for evaluating these competencies and the effectiveness of various programs.

Promoting Personal and Interpersonal Communication

Personal communication and interpersonal communication were also defined as basic skills that are essential for customer and service orientation as well as for teamwork and working with clients (Jarva et al., 2023; Maeda & Socha-Dietrich, 2021). Communication between caregivers and patients has been recognized as an important component in treatment encounters. Effective communication promotes relations and trust between caregivers and patients, influences patient satisfaction, increases patients' desire to respond to treatment and even improves clinical indexes and safety during treatment (King & Hoppe, 2013). Over the past decades, nursing and medical schools have introduced numerous programs to teach interpersonal communication skills, with emphasis on patient-caregiver relationships. Among other things, students learn and practice communication in clinical settings, active listening, and conducting medical interviews while taking the patient's personal and cultural characteristics into consideration. Models such as the Calgary-Cambridge Model (Kurtz et al., 2003) and the Kalamazoo Model (Makoul, 2001) are becoming more widely accepted and used.

The Calgary–Cambridge model was developed by experts from the Faculty of Medicine at the University of Cambridge and the University of Calgary, Canada. This consultation model defines five stages that successively replace each other (consultation opening; information gathering; review; explanation and planning; and consultation conclusion). Each stage includes tasks that must be solved using certain skills. Moreover, two ongoing processes run from the beginning to the end of the consultation (structuring and building a trusting relationship). These models are used to enable students to practice clinical exposure in hospitals or in the community (Finkelstein et al., 2019). Students engage in simulation and role-playing games with actors (e.g., standardized patients), and their interactions are videotaped and analyzed. Training using simulation is currently accepted as one of the effective ways to develop interpersonal communication skills. Indeed, simulation enables students to gain abilities and practical experience in conducting interviews and to receive professional feedback (Henriksen et al., 2018; Markin et al., 2015).

Nurturing Empathy Among Students

Several models are also used in various courses to teach medical students to develop communication competency and empathy. One such models is the SPINKES Model (Meitar et al., 2009), which is used to teach students to convey difficult news to patients. Other models enable students to practice communal decision-making (Karnieli-Miller et al., 2014). These models have become an integral part of medical humanities education—a field that aims to assimilate social sciences such as sociology, anthropology and psychology into medical education. This approach supports the notion that medical studies should provide a broad perspective on patients and their illnesses, one that includes the patients' families, communities and cultural and political environment. This broader patient perspective, along with a focus on their wellbeing, will enhance the communication and empathy abilities of medical staff personnel in the future (Bleakley et al., 2013).

Implementing Customer Service Through Guidance and Workshops

Other reviewed programs dealt with the assimilation of management processes in hospitals, for example through guidance and simulation workshops that cover basic customer service principles, recognizing patients as customers, service industry benchmarking leaders, stress recognition, communication skills, negotiation skills, proactive customer service, change management, and specific customer service core competencies. In addition, customer service workshops offer annual updates on conflict resolution, customer service and communication skills, and assertiveness training.

Most education programs geared to developing the competencies needed to achieve change and promote a service orientation are offered at the personal level during training and are designed to train students before they join the workforce. Teaching these topics during the early stages of training has gained additional validity based on studies showing that workers who already possess high levels of service orientation have a hiring advantage. The effectiveness of attempting to develop these traits among workers at a later stage is unclear (O'Connor et al., 2000).

Today many institutions engaged in training medical personnel are required to assimilate humanitarian medical education. Nevertheless, these programs are not uniform, either in their content or in their evaluation indexes. Moreover, there is a shortage of instructors capable of linking these topics to the medical field (Finkelstein et al., 2019). This program variance contrasts sharply with the scientific clinical aspects of medical studies, which are governed by national standards in assessment and issuing medical licenses. While humanitarian education has traditionally appeared to be vague and open to the whims of various individuals within training institutions, lacking supervision (Schwartz et al., 2009), the incorporation of health humanities is increasingly gaining traction. This trend supports the work of integrating a broader, more structured approach to humanitarian education in medical training (Bleakley, 2023).

In addition, researchers called upon to assess the long-term influence of humanistic studies must find empirical as well as non-quantitative methodological tools suitable for evaluating these complex educational processes (Finkelstein et al., 2019).

Discussion

In recent decades, change processes at the personal level have become an integral part of the clinical side of professional medical and nursing training (Finkelstein et al., 2019). Nevertheless, these change processes still need to be assimilated at the meso and macro levels, and organizational and system management and leadership need to be trained in the necessary skills (Naamati-Schneider, 2023).

Alongside learning to develop these competencies, medical staff members at all levels of the system need to be trained in the communication skills necessary for promoting a digital service orientation. Managerial and medical staff members are currently voicing objections to the digital technology being assimilated in the system as part of the change process. The difficulties encountered by workers at all levels present obstacles that hinder them in adopting these change processes. For this reason, tailor-made training in these technologies together with training in how to use digital tools and acquire digital skills are essential to eliminate opposition and phobias, while placing emphasis on general service skills (De Leeuw et al., 2020; Jarva et al., 2023; Maeda & Socha-Dietrich, 2021). There is no doubt that a service orientation requires a broad and comprehensive vision at all levels of the organization. The healthcare system must focus on customers/patients while retaining a service-centered and client-centered orientation. Rapid technological advances will require workers to acquire a variety of technological and service-orientation skills, as well as to meet constantly growing and complex demands (Jolanki et al., 2017; Vehko et al., 2019). Medical education and instruction must be integrated with the acquisition of skills and competencies such as communication, empathy, teamwork, and cooperation in mixed teams. Indeed, a multi-cultural vision is essential for assimilating an all-embracing service-orientation, in conjunction with processes for applying assimilated digital technologies. In this way the healthcare system, its organizations, its managers and its medical staff will be able to make the transition to a service orientation.

We therefore recommend expanding these areas of learning and assimilating the acquisition of these skills at all levels of the system, from the first stages of training to professional training and throughout the careers of managers and caregivers at all levels. Thus, the organization will be able to assimilate a strong organizational culture that integrates all aspects of the organization, including treatment and service procedures, based on empathy, as part of the organization's transition to a client and service orientation. The ultimate result will be a high-quality, modern, service-oriented and sustainable system that will benefit both customers and service providers.

Adopting a uniform and integrative approach to developing these capabilities across the entire system is essential for creating a single uniform language among all training institutions and during all stages of training, beginning at the early stages and continuing throughout training and workers' professional lives. Developing and assimilating these programs is expected to be fraught with difficulties and problems. Human and financial resources as well as research will be needed to develop and assess intervention programs and examine their long-term effectiveness and benefits. Such programs will also require people who are able to teach these skills and apply them in organizational practice within the healthcare system. Training staff members in this area demands extensive multidisciplinary vision as well as allotting resources to implement these challenges. Meeting and implementing these challenges will ensure the sustainability and quality of the study content as well as long-term assimilation of the changes. Additionally, an organizational structure and support that reflect that health professionals should focus on the wellbeing of all is essential. The ultimate goal is to ensure the creation of service- and customer-oriented healthcare systems, while utilizing resources in a correct, effective, and sustainable manner.

References

Aka Zohar, A. (2019). Eichut be-mifgash metapel metupal: Tfisa hadasha (Quality in the encounter between clinician and patient: A new approach). In S. Shafran-Sigal, Y. Shemer, & Y. Weiss (Eds.), *Mifgashim be'olam habriut (Encounters in the world of health)* (pp. 235–272). Akademon [in Hebrew].

Ampaw, E. M., Liang, B., Tsai, S. B., & Frempong, J. (2020). Assessment on health care service quality and patients' satisfaction in Ghana. *Kybernetes, 49*(12), 3047–3068.

Attree, M. (2001). Patients' and relatives' experiences and perspectives of 'good' and 'not so good' quality care. *The Journal of Advanced Nursing* (*JAN*), *33*, 4. https://doi.org/10.1046/j.1365-2648.2001.01689.x

Birk, R. (2019). Tikshoret ba-tzevet ha-refu'ui ba-idan ha-digitali: Kli hiuni le-tipul ba-metupal (Communication in the medical team in the digital age: An essential tool in patient care). In S. Shafran-Sigal, Y. Shemer, & Y. Weiss (Eds.), *Mifgashim be'olam habriut (Encounters in the world of health)* (pp. 129–139). Akademon [Hebrew].

Bleakley, A. (2023). *Medical humanities: Ethics, aesthetics, politics*. Taylor & Francis.

Bleakley, A., & Marshall, R. (2013). Can the science of communication inform the art of the medical humanities? *Medical Education, 47*(2), 126–133. https://doi.org/10.1111/medu.12056

Chang, C. S., Chen, S. Y., & Lan, Y. T. (2013). Service quality, trust, and patient satisfaction in interpersonal-based medical service encounters. *BMC Health Services Research, 22*, 1472–6963.

De Leeuw, J. A., Woltjer, H., & Kool, R. B. (2020). Identification of factors influencing the adoption of health information technology by nurses who are digitally lagging: In-depth interview study. *Journal Medical Internet Resources, 22*(8), e15630. https://doi.org/10.2196/15630

Denis, J. L., & van Gestel, N. (2015). Leadership and innovation in healthcare governance. In E. Kuhlmann, R. H. Blank, I. L. Bourgeault, & C. Wendt (Eds.), *The Palgrave international handbook of healthcare policy and governance* (pp. 425–440). Palgrave Macmillan. https://doi.org/10.1057/9781137384935_26

Dolev, N., Naamati-Schneider, L., & Meirovich, A. (2021). *Making soft skills a part of the curriculum of healthcare studies*. IntechOpen

Dreiher, D., Blagorazumnaya, O., Balicer, R., et al. (2020). National initiatives to promote quality of care and patient safety: Achievements to date and challenges ahead. *Israel Journal Health Policy Research, 9*, 62. https://doi.org/10.1186/s13584-020-00417-x

Endeshaw, B. (2021). Healthcare service quality-measurement models: A review. *Journal of Health Research, 35*(2), 106–117. https://doi.org/10.1108/JHR-07-2019-0152

Erkan, I., & Mehmet, U. N. A. L. (2022) Total quality management practices in health services. *Research Journal of Business and Management, 9*(4), 197–205.

Fenton, J. J., Jerant, A. F., Bertakis, K. D., & Franks, P. (2012). The cost of satisfaction: A national study of patient satisfaction, health care utilization, expenditures, and mortality. *Archives of Internal Medicine, 172*(5), 405–411. https://doi.org/10.1001/archinternmed.2011.1662

Finkelstein, A., Kraniaeli Miller, O., Meitar, D., & Orkin, Y. (2019). Humanistic education in medicine and its implementation in medical schools in Israel. In S. Shafran-Tikva, Y. Shamir, & Y. Weiss (Eds.), *Encounters in the world of health* (pp. 73–89). Academon. [In Hebrew].

Gilbert, P., & Laporte, M.-E. (2023). Patient orientation in public hospitals: A marketing device as compromise between worlds. *Recherche et Applications En Marketing (English Edition)*. https://doi-org.mgs.hac.ac.il/10.1177/20515707221146485

Gong, Z., Chen, Y., & Wang, Y. (2019). The influence of emotional intelligence on job burnout and job performance: mediating effect of psychological capital. *Frontiers in Psychology, 10*, 2707. https://doi.org/10.3389/fpsyg.2019.02707

Groene, O., Lombarts, M. J. M. H., Klazinga, N., Alonso, J., Thompson, A., & Suñol, R. (2009). Is patient-centredness in European hospitals related to existing quality improvement strategies? Analysis of a cross-sectional survey (MARQuIS study). *BMJ Quality and Safety, 18*(Suppl 1), i44–i50. https://doi.org/10.1136/qshc.2008.029397

Halvorsen, B., Bartram, T., Kia, N., & Cavanagh, J. (2023). Meeting customer needs through ethical leadership and training: Examining Australian bank employees. *Asia Pacific Journal of Human Resources, 61*(1), 79–100. https://doi-org.mgs.hac.ac.il/10.1111/1744-7941.12329

Henrike, H.-W., & Schultz, C. (2014). The impact of health care professionals' service orientation on patients' innovative behavior. *Health Care Management Review, 39*(4), 329–339. https://www.jstor.org/stable/48516403

Henriksen, K., Rodrick, D., Grace, E. N., & Brady, P. J. (2018). Challenges in health care simulation: Are we learning anything new? *Academic Medicine, 93*(5), 705–708. https://doi.org/10.1097/ACM.0000000000001891

Hogan, J., Hogan, R., & Busch, C. M. (1984). How to measure service orientation. *Journal of Applied Psychology, 69*(1), 167–173. https://doi.org/10.1037/0021-9010.69.1.167

Jarva, E., Oikarinen, A., Andersson, J., Tomietto, M., Kääriäinen, M., & Mikkonen, K. (2023). Healthcare professionals' digital health competence and its core factors; development and psychometric testing of two instruments. *International Journal of Medical Informatics*, 104995. https://doi.org/10.1016/j.ijmedinf.2023.104995

Jolanki, O., Tynkkynen, L., & Sinervo, T. (2017). Professionals' views on integrated care. *Journal of Integrated Care*. https://doi.org/10.1108/JICA-06-2017-0018

Jongen, C., McCalman, J., Bainbridge, R., Clifford, A. (2018a). Health workforce development interventions to improve cultural competence. In *Cultural competence in health. Springer briefs in public health*. Springer. https://doi-org.mgs.hac.ac.il/10.1007/978-981-10-5293-4_4

Jongen, C., McCalman, J. & Bainbridge, R. (2018b). Health workforce cultural competency interventions: a systematic scoping review. *BMC Health Service Resources, 18*, 232. https://doi-org.mgs.hac.ac.il/10.1186/s12913-018-3001-5

Karnieli-Miller, O., Zisman-Ilani, Y., Meitar, D., & Mekori, Y. (2014). The role of medical schools in promoting social accountability through shared decision-making. *Israel Journal of Health Policy Research, 3*(1), 1–4. https://doi.org/10.1186/2045-4015-3-26

King, A., & Hoppe, R. B. (2013). Best practice for patient-centered communication: A narrative review. *Journal of Graduate Medical Education, 5*(3), 385–393. https://doi.org/10.4300/JGME-D-13-00072.1

Kraus, S., Schiavone, F., Pluzhnikova, A., & Invernizzi, A. C. (2021). Digital transformation in healthcare: Analyzing the current state-of-research. *Journal of Business Research, 123*, 557–567. https://doi.org/10.1016/j.jbusres.2020.10.030

Kurtz, S., Silverman, J., Benson, J., & Draper, J. (2003). Marrying content and process in clinical method teaching: Enhancing the Calgary-Cambridge guides. *Academic Medicine, 78*(8), 802–809.

Lagrosen, S., & Lagrosen, Y. (2022). Workplace stress and health–the connection to quality management. *Total Quality Management and Business Excellence, 33*(1–2), 113–126. https://doi.org/10.1080/14783363.2020.1807317

Maeda, K., & Socha-Dietrich, K. (2021). Skills for the future health workforce: Preparing health professionals for people-centred care. *OECD Health Working Papers, 124*. https://doi.org/10.1787/68fb5f08-en

Makoul, G. (2001). Essential elements of communication in medical encounters: The Kalamazoo consensus statement. *Academic Medicine, 76*(4), 390–393. https://doi.org/10.1155/2015/534879

Markin, A., Cabrera-Fernandez, D. F., Bajoka, R. M., Noll, S. M., Drake, S. M., Awdish, R. L., Buick, D. S., Kokas, M. S., Chasteen, K. A., & Mendez, M. P. (2015). Impact of a simulation-based communication workshop on resident preparedness for end-of-life communication in the intensive care unit. *Critical Care Research and Practice*. https://doi.org/10.1155/2015/534879

Marques, I. C. P., & Ferreira, J. J. M. (2020). Digital transformation in the area of health: Systematic review of 45 years of evolution. *Health and Technology, 10*(3), 575–586.

Meitar, D., Karnieli-Miller, O., & Eidelman, S. (2009). The impact of senior medical students' personal difficulties on their communication patterns in breaking bad news. *Academic Medicine, 84*(11), 1582–1594. https://doi.org/10.1097/ACM.0b013e3181bb2b94

Naamati-Schneider, L. (2020). Strategic management as adaptation to changes in the ecosystems of public hospitals in Israel. *Israel Journal Health Policy Research, 9*, 65. https://doi.org/10.1186/s13584-020-00424-y

Naamati-Schneider, L. (2021). Public-private: Unequal competition Israeli public hospitals vs the private health-care system following government reforms. *International Journal of Organizational Analysis, 29*(6), 1381–1394. https://doi.org/10.1108/IJOA-06-2020-2237

Naamati-Schneider, L. (2022). Intraorganisation conflicts of interest in hospitals adapting to a changing ecosystem. *Journal of Health Organisation and Management*. https://doi.org/10.1108/jhom-09-2021-0325

Naamati-Schneider, L. (2023). The effect of digitalization on service orientation and service perception among Israeli healthcare professionals: A qualitative study. *Digital Health, 9*, 20552076231191892.

Naamati-Schneider, L., Salvatore, F. P. (2023). Sustainability for healthcare organisations and systems: cultivating strategy and governance processes for a better future. In D. Vrontis, A. Thrassou, L. Efthymiou, Y. Weber, S. M. R. Shams, & E. Tsoukatos (Eds.), *Business for sustainability, Volume I. Palgrave studies in cross-disciplinary business research, in association with EuroMed Academy of Business*. Palgrave Macmillan. https://doi.org/10.1007/978-3-031-37361-9_11

Naamati-Schneider, L., & Zaks O. (2022) Public hospitals in crisis: Managerial and strategic adaptation. In D. Vrontis, A. Thrassou, Y. Weber, S. M. R. Shams, E. Tsoukatos, L. Efthymiou (Eds.), *Business under crisis, Volume II. Palgrave studies in cross-disciplinary business research, in association with EuroMed Academy of Business*. Palgrave Macmillan. https://doi.org/10.1007/978-3-030-76575-0_3

O'Connor, S. J., Trinh, H. Q., & Shewchuk, R. M. (2000). Determinants of service orientation among medical students. In *Advances in health care management* (Vol. 1, pp. 217–249). Emerald Group Publishing Limited. https://doi.org/10.1016/S1474-8231(00)01010-7

Patricio, L., Sangiorgi, D., Mahr, D., Čaić, M., Kalantari, S., & Sundar, S. (2020). Leveraging service design for healthcare transformation: Toward people-centered, integrated, and technology-enabled healthcare systems. *Journal of Service Management, 31*(5), 889–909. https://doi-org.mgs.hac.ac.il/10.1108/JOSM-11-2019-0332

Porter, M. E., & Lee, T. H. (2016). From volume to value in health care: The work begins. *JAMA, 316*(10), 1047–1048.

Powers, T. L., & Bendall, D. (2004). Improving health outcomes through patient empowerment. *Journal of Hospital Marketing and Public Relations, 15*(1), 45–59. https://doi.org/10.2139/ssrn.2140763

Präg, P., Wittek, R., & Mills, M. C. (2017). The educational gradient in self-rated health in Europe: Does the doctor–patient relationship make a difference? *Acta Sociologica, 60*(4), 325–341. https://doi.org/10.1177/0001699316670715

Richards, T., Montori, V. M., Godlee, F., Lapsley, P., & Paul, D. (2013). Let the patient revolution begin. *BMJ, 346*. https://doi.org/10.1136/bmj.f2614

Roe, Y. L., Zeitz, C. J., & Fredericks, B. (2012). Study protocol: Establishing good relationships between patients and health care providers while providing cardiac care. Exploring how patient-clinician engagement contributes to health disparities between indigenous and non-indigenous Australians in South Australia. *BMC Health Service Resources, 12*(1), 1–10.

Schwartz, A. W., Abramson, J. S., Wojnowich, I., Accordino, R., Ronan, E. J., & Rifkin, M. R. (2009). Evaluating the impact of the humanities in medical education. *Mount Sinai Journal of Medicine: A Journal of Translational and Personalized Medicine: A Journal of Translational and Personalized Medicine, 76*(4), 372–380. https://doi.org/10.1002/msj.20126

Serrat, O. (2017). Understanding and developing emotional intelligence. In *Knowledge Solutions*. Springer. https://doi.org/10.1007/978-981-10-0983-9_37

Shaller, D. (2007). *Patient-centered care: What does it take?* (pp. 1–26). Commonwealth Fund.

Singh, K. (2012). Enhancing service orientation through emotional intelligence amongst health care professionals: A case study of government hospital in Delhi, India. *India*. https://doi.org/10.2139/ssrn.2140763

Sriatmi, A., Jati, S. P., & Fatmasari, E. Y. (2020). The influence of organizational factors on compliance with the standard planning process in primary health care. *Journal of Public Health for Tropical and Coastal Region, 3*(1), 9–16. https://doi.org/10.14710/jphtcr.v3i1.7531

Truong, M., Paradies, Y., & Priest, N. (2014). Interventions to improve cultural competency in healthcare: A systematic review of reviews. *BMC Health Services Research, 14*, 99. https://doi.org/10.1186/1472-6963-14-99

Tung, W., Liang, A., & Chen, S. C. (2014). The influence of service orientation and interaction orientation on consumer identification. *The Service Industries Journal, 34*(5), 439–454. https://doi.org/10.1080/02642069.2014.871533

Vaish, A., Vaish, A., Vaishya, R., & Bhawal, A. (2016). Customer relationship management (CRM) towards service orientation in hospitals: A review. *Apollo Medicine, 13*(4), 224–228. https://doi.org/10.1016/j.apme.2016.11.002

Vehko, T., Hyppönen, H., Puttonen, S., et al. (2019). Experienced time pressure and stress: Electronic health records usability and information technology competence play a role. *BMC Medical Informatics and Decision Making, 19*, 160. https://doi.org/10.1186/s12911-019-0891-z

Vyas, S., Bhargava, D., & Khan, S. (2023). Healthcare 4.0: A systematic review and its impact over conventional healthcare system. *Artificial Intelligence for Health 4.0: Challenges and Applications*, 1–17.

Yang, J. H., & Yoon, J. A. (2023). Comparative analysis of the effect of job satisfaction on customer oriented behaviors by personality type of nurses. *Journal for ReAttach Therapy and Developmental Diversities, 6*(1s), 01–12.

Zhang, L., Tong, H., Demirel, H. O., Duffy, V. G., Yih, Y., & Bidassie, B. (2015). A practical model of value co-creation in healthcare service. *Procedia Manufacturing, 3*, 200–207. https://doi.org/10.1016/j.promfg.2015.07.129

Chapter 11
Online Collaborative Padlet-Mediated Learning in Health Management Studies

Abstract Developing collaboration skills is imperative for healthcare professionals, and early integration of online collaborative learning (OCL) methodologies cultivates these essential competencies. This chapter illustrates the efficacy of OCL through the use of Padlet in health management education. It highlights the significant benefits of adopting OCL methodologies for the healthcare system and its patients. By analyzing students' experiences with Padlet, the chapter emphasizes its role in enhancing teamwork, decision-making abilities, and adaptability. These findings underscore Padlet's transformative impact in preparing healthcare professionals for dynamic, collaborative settings.

Introduction

This chapter illustrates the effectiveness of online collaborative learning (OCL) as a teaching method for health management students. Specifically, the chapter examines the use of Padlet as a digital platform for interactive collaboration. Acquisition of collaboration skills is crucial for health professionals, who often work in multidisciplinary and culturally diverse teams. These skills can be developed by exposing students to online collaborative learning (OCL) environments early in their professional training (Männistö et al., 2020). The adoption and advancement of OCL pedagogies across all levels of education, from undergraduate studies to professional development, is widely believed to benefit both the health system and its patients by enabling healthcare workers to meet the demands of the healthcare market. OCL is particularly relevant in light of the practical nature of work in the health industry (Grosser et al., 2020).

This chapter analyzes students' perspectives regarding their experiences using Padlet-enabled OCL. It seeks to understand how the students perceived the Padlet activity and its implications. Content analysis was used to help identify themes and patterns regarding students' perceptions of the newly designed activity. The chapter focuses on understanding the benefits of Padlet as a collaborative learning tool so as to

L. Naamati-Schneider and D. Alt, *Technology and Competency-Oriented Learning*,
https://doi.org/10.1007/978-981-97-5771-8_11

develop students' ability to work in diverse teams, to collaborate in decision-making, and to adapt to changes in the learning environment.

In this section we review the advantages as well as the challenges of OCL. We also address Padlet-mediated learning in technology-enhanced environments by reviewing relevant recent literature. Further, we describe the use of this teaching methodology in the healthcare professions and examine its impact on the skills required of today's healthcare students.

Online Collaborative Learning

Zheng et al. (2014) defined online collaborative learning (OCL) as a goal-oriented activity carried out by a group of students committed to achieving a shared goal and to creating new knowledge through interactive learning in a digital environment. This methodology has become widespread because of its many advantages. For example, studies have shown that encouragement of student engagement, high accessibility to course material (Balouchi & Samad, 2021; Sukendro et al., 2020), extensive access to colleagues and instructors, and encouragement of interaction and collaboration among students contribute to better learning outcomes. OCL was found to add interest and to increase motivation for research and study. As such, it encourages the transition from passive to active learning and fosters interaction and connection between students by sharing the products of their study and new ideas. All of this results in greater social engagement and contributes to the development of higher-order intellectual skills (Park et al., 2019; Yadegaridehkordi et al., 2019).

Various studies (Ng et al., 2022) have explored the factors affecting the degree to which students adopt OCL. For example, Cole et al. (2021) showed that students' perceptions of the online learning environment were an important factor in predicting their engagement in learning by means of online courses. Qureshi et al. (2023) identified the following key factors in the degree of OCL adoption and the extent to which it influences achievement of learning goals and improved performance: nature of the social interaction in the learning environment, support and positive interaction with the facilitator, and type of technology used. Other studies evaluated the level and quality of OCL outcomes. DiPasquale (2017), for example, discussed ways of evaluating OCL outcomes by analyzing the use of brainstorming, group discussion, and oral and written presentation of ideas during the initial stages of establishing higher-order learning outcomes. Blieck et al. (2019) noted that this methodology promoted the development and encouragement of ideas as outcomes of higher-order learning and cited the guidance and support provided by the instructor. Similarly, Aldholay et al. (2018) demonstrated how students developed higher-order thinking while processing, reflecting on, and analyzing collaborative critical thinking about specific topics relevant to course content. Such a supportive and collaborative learning environment facilitates the emergence of an effective learning perspective for attaining maximum learning goals.

Online Collaborative Learning Mediated by Padlet

The Padlet interactive platform serves as a virtual online bulletin board on which users can post various types of multimedia content, such as documents, questions, comments, images, video clips, and audio clips. The platform and the board are available to learners throughout their studies and even afterwards (Mehta et al., 2021). Recent studies have shown that Padlet-mediated learning has been effective in encouraging learners through active teaching and collaborative learning (Rashid et al., 2019).

According to a study by Gasmi and Thomas (2017), the Padlet technology promotes collaboration among learners together with student engagement in seminar courses. The study found that the technology helped make students' studies more effective and provided an easy and secure learning environment for communication, teamwork, and asking questions. All these studies view the use of Padlet-mediated collaborative learning in a positive light by citing the tool's advantages: ease of use, accessibility to materials over time (even after the course is over), and use of diverse resources (including links, images, and video clips), thus making it a convenient tool for student-focused active collaborative learning (Mehta et al., 2021).

Several studies have demonstrated the benefits of using Padlet as a tool for collaborative learning. For example, Beltrán-Martín (2019) reported satisfaction and improved academic performance among students who used the platform. Padlet's identified advantages for collaborative learning include ease of use, long-term content accessibility, and ability to incorporate a range of resources, such as presentations, links, images, and videos. These features offer a holistic and student-centered approach to teaching and learning, as students are able to use their preferred medium and become actively involved in creating their own content.

Nevertheless, a review of the literature also indicates that Padlet-mediated OCL methodologies are not yet widely used in higher education, particularly in the fields of medical education and medical management. Moreover, very little research has examined how these methodologies are used in higher education. This chapter showcases how an intervention program that incorporated Padlet-mediated OCL can be used in health management studies. Furthermore, the chapter evaluates the program's effectiveness in promoting collaborative learning by examining the perspectives of 85 Israeli undergraduate students enrolled in a health management program. Tracing student engagement in online learning activities (as opposed to face-to-face learning encounters) is difficult, especially in studies that examine students' perspectives. Hence, in order to understand the effects of using this technology-mediated methodology for achieving learning goals and acquiring the requisite skills, it is essential to map students' perceptions. The data from such studies can help in evaluating the effectiveness of this learning methodology (Mehta et al., 2021).

The students in our test case were asked to keep a reflective journal throughout the course and submit it at the end of the semester. They were instructed to record their impressions of the learning process by describing their main challenges, difficulties, and positive and negative experiences. In the journals the students were able to reflect on significant learning processes and adopt a multidimensional view of them (Alt et al., 2022).

Instructional Method Procedure: Padlet-Mediated OCL

In this case study, we converted a required course titled Introducing Quality into the Health System taught using a traditional frontal format into a course that used Padlet-mediated OCL methodology (Naamati-Schneider & Alt, 2023a, 2023b). The methodology facilitated OCL in the following ways: working in small groups; building a collaborative data pool; carrying out final projects that focused on dilemmas and analyzing these dilemmas in organizations using a student-constructed data pool; presenting the projects on collaborative platforms; and peer review (Ng et al., 2022). At the beginning of the course, the students were exposed to the new teaching method and instructed how to use the Padlet technology. The technology was further demonstrated when the method was introduced through presentations of students using the Padlet board. This introduction helped students become familiar with the tool, thus providing them with informal and equal experience using the tool and generating student interactions to create groups and increase student engagement in the course (Qureshi et al., 2023).

The course consisted of several stages, each based on the one that preceded it. After becoming familiar with the course outline and technology, the students were asked to form online study groups in which they would work throughout the semester. In the second stage, the students were asked to choose a topic from among the course topics listed on the Padlet board. In the following stage, the study groups were asked to formulate a question, problem, or dilemma related to the selected topic and to gather information from articles on the topic. They were then asked to describe and analyze the articles in the context of the selected topic and to post their conclusions on a new Padlet board, which was organized by topics and subtopics. Topics selected included dilemmas in instituting accreditation processes, challenges in maintaining medical confidentiality, clinician-patient relationships maintained by digital tools, and assessment of an organization's quality of service.

This stage ended with the creation of a categorical board containing information, articles, and links to academic content. This categorical board constituted a collaborative information bank that was congruent with the course topics and categorically divided for easy navigation and accessibility by all the students in all the groups (Mehta et al., 2021). In the next stage, the groups were asked to prepare and present a final project, which was posted on yet another Padlet board. This project, which was based on the preceding work, required students to extend the scope of the original project into a comprehensive research question or discussion of a specific dilemma in a particular organization. The objective was to include a number of perspectives that among other things were based on the collaborative knowledge pool of the entire class, and even to extend the project by adding new materials.

As part of the final project, the students were required to provide organizational and managerial perspectives as well as the perspectives of patients and health professionals. They were instructed to accomplish this by means of online group meetings and collaborative work, including brainstorming, discussion, and decision-making regarding how the final project would be constructed and visually presented on a Padlet board. They had the option of choosing among various formats and using different technologies, including, for example, e-posters, presentations, and video clips created by technologies such as PowerPoint and ThingLink, which they had learned in other courses. The option to use various technologies empowered individual students by allowing freedom of choice in how to present their conclusions, constituting an advantage of the Padlet technology. The third board brought together all the projects in the course. The students were required to use the Padlet board to critique the projects their classmates exhibited on that board, ask questions, add information, or highlight topics to be added to the discussion of the dilemma. Table 11.1 summarizes the procedure used in the instructional method.

Thematic analysis was used to identify and report on topics that emerged from the data. Each theme was summarized to provide an overview of the participants' reports. The dominant topics in the reflective journals were then identified and gathered together as main categories.

Students' Perceptions of Padlet-Mediated OCL

The data analysis of the reflective journals revealed seven main categories, as indicated in Fig. 11.1. Exemplary quotes from the data are provided to illustrate each category.

User Experience with the Platform

Analysis of the students' journals revealed that the students found using the interface easy and positive. Most of them indicated that using the platform did not require much learning and experience, stating that after a relatively brief explanation they were able to use it freely. Hence, the platform makes the user experience easy and pleasant.

> It was very easy in my opinion, and therefore also made them [the Padlet assignments] very enjoyable. They were almost easier and more enjoyable than all the other assignments in other courses.

Many of the students stated that for them, using the platform was almost as experiential as using social media and other familiar and favorite applications they use for online social interaction. This gave them confidence in using a familiar and informal tool, thus reducing their resistance and anxiety in carrying out their assignments.

Table 11.1 Instructional method procedure

Program stages	Students' role	Instructor's role	Learning outcomes
Stage 1	1. Self-introduction on the Padlet board	1. Presenting the technologies and requirements 2. Self-introduction	Introductory Padlet board—learning about the platform and about fellow students
Stage 2	1. Choosing one of the presented situations 2. Identifying and defining the dilemma. Discussing how the perspectives are reflected in the dilemma and choosing one perspective	1. Presenting the dilemmas 2. Describing the assignment: choosing a situation and constructing the dilemma. Providing technical explanations about how to use the Padlet board	Padlet Board 1—situations and dilemmas
Stage 3	1. Searching for relevant information 2. Presenting topic-related articles and paper abstracts	1. Teaching the course content, including the dilemmas and their applications and consequences 2. Explaining the triple relationship between healthcare provider, patient, and organization	Padlet Board 2—a shared knowledge base divided into categories and perspectives
Stage 4	1. Using databases to build the final project 2. Presenting the final project on Padlet 3. Examining peers' work and giving feedback	1. Guiding students in the final project 2. Examining the projects and giving feedback	Padlet Board 3—Final projects
During and after the learning	Writing a reflective journal in which students examine their personal learning process during the stages and describe the experiences, opportunities, and challenges posed by the learning in general and the use of Padlet in particular. Journals were voluntarily submitted at the end of the process	In this study, students were asked general questions, such as "describe your experience during the learning process." They could address these questions in their journals, as well as in freestyle writing that allowed open-ended reflection	Reflective journal—average length 1000–1500 words, about 7–8 paragraphs

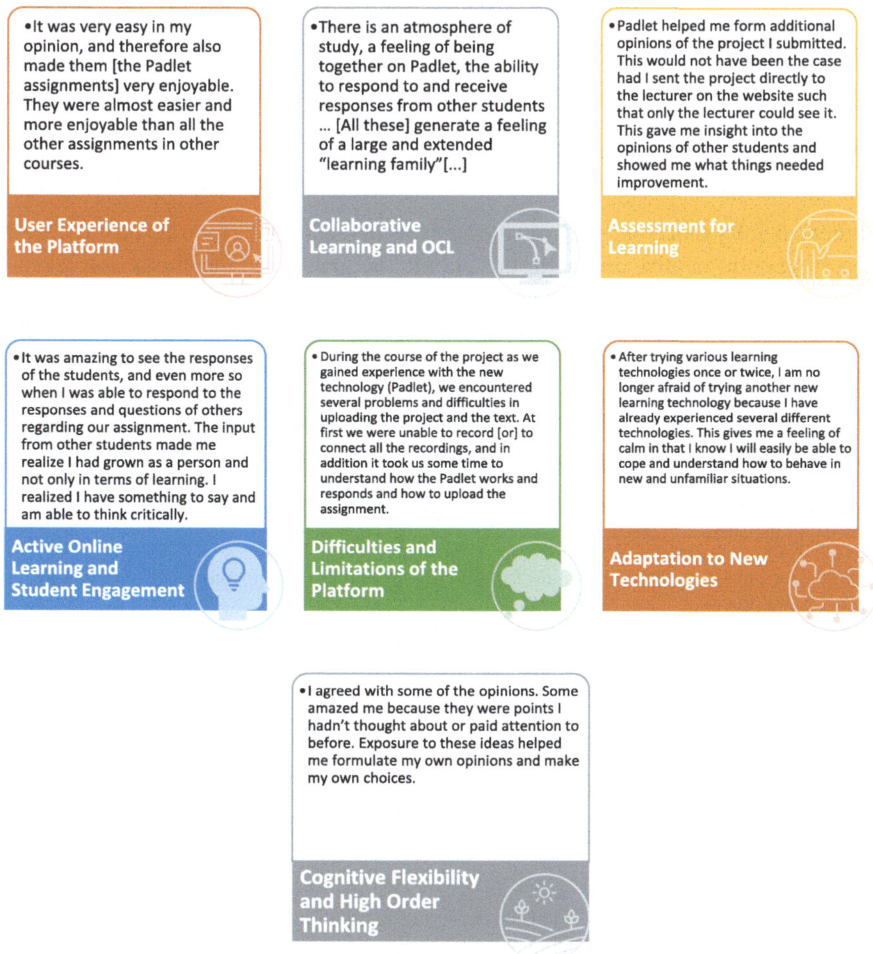

•It was very easy in my opinion, and therefore also made them [the Padlet assignments] very enjoyable. They were almost easier and more enjoyable than all the other assignments in other courses.
User Experience of the Platform
•There is an atmosphere of study, a feeling of being together on Padlet, the ability to respond to and receive responses from other students ... [All these] generate a feeling of a large and extended "learning family"[...]
Collaborative Learning and OCL
•Padlet helped me form additional opinions of the project I submitted. This would not have been the case had I sent the project directly to the lecturer on the website such that only the lecturer could see it. This gave me insight into the opinions of other students and showed me what things needed improvement.
Assessment for Learning
•It was amazing to see the responses of the students, and even more so when I was able to respond to the responses and questions of others regarding our assignment. The input from other students made me realize I had grown as a person and not only in terms of learning. I realized I have something to say and am able to think critically.
Active Online Learning and Student Engagement
•During the course of the project as we gained experience with the new technology (Padlet), we encountered several problems and difficulties in uploading the project and the text. At first we were unable to record [or] to connect all the recordings, and in addition it took us some time to understand how the Padlet works and responds and how to upload the assignment.
Difficulties and Limitations of the Platform
•After trying various learning technologies once or twice, I am no longer afraid of trying another new learning technology because I have already experienced several different technologies. This gives me a feeling of calm in that I know I will easily be able to cope and understand how to behave in new and unfamiliar situations.
Adaptation to New Technologies
•I agreed with some of the opinions. Some amazed me because they were points I hadn't thought about or paid attention to before. Exposure to these ideas helped me formulate my own opinions and make my own choices.
Cognitive Flexibility and High Order Thinking

Fig. 11.1 Derived categories and exemplary quotes from the data

> I think this is very similar to Facebook, and all kinds of social media that are more attractive to us, the "young' public. Lots of posts for enriching information or nice bits that you read and, by the way, also learn.

Several students made positive comments about the platform's visual presentation and the fact that it can be changed according to students' and instructors' preferences. For example, the instructor was able to determine the background and organization of the Padlet, while each group was able choose the format for adding materials.

> I assumed responsibility for posting the summary on Padlet. I enjoyed doing that because the platform offered all kinds of possibilities for inserting our personality in the arrangement and colors and highlights. After I organized everything… I decided we should make a video

clip briefly describing our work. This was really fun and interesting and unique No one else did anything similar.

Collaborative Learning and OCL

Another category that emerged from the analysis of the journals focused on OCL, i.e., on creating collaborative online groups at both the **group** and the **classroom** levels. **The group level** encompassed activities that required teamwork within the group: creating the pool, preparing the assignments, and posting the assignments on the board. According to the students, these assignments included information sharing, brainstorming, and decision-making, with the aim of producing group output as required by the assignment. Analysis of the journals revealed a strong feeling of collaboration among the group members.

> [The use of Padlet] strengthened the ties among the members of the project team. We thought about all the sections together, considered how to argue, and so on.

> I felt we were all together and could follow each other and respond and receive ideas and think more deeply.

At class level, the collaborative learning experience extended beyond the close circle of group members needed to present a project using the Padlet platform. Despite the large number of students, the collaboration also included the other students in the course. Indeed, the fact that this tool can be used effectively even in very large groups was considered an advantage in that project presentation via Padlet is not limited by the number of students or by time.

> There is an atmosphere of study, a feeling of being together on Padlet, the ability to respond to and receive responses from other students … [All these] generate a feeling of a large and extended "learning family". This empowering feeling [was] so important and significant during the COVID-19 pandemic, which over the past two year has created a sense of loneliness and alienation and disrupted the learning atmosphere.

Nevertheless, in their reflective journals many students noted their initial concerns about posting material related to class assignments. They explained this concern based on their previous experience in which other students often copied material from them. Several students described their perceptual transition from individual, even competitive, learning to a collaborative perception of shared knowledge and ideas that were mutually developed and inspired, constituting a stage in processing knowledge and a great source of personal development.

> For me personally I was a bit concerned that perhaps other students would copy my ideas and take advantage of the situation, but very quickly I understood that this was not possible, Moreover, students responded to me all the way… In truth, I was surprised to see this happening. The thought that someone might copy my ideas is really off-putting.

Some students also expressed fears related to collaboration. These were primarily students who feared criticism, had low self-confidence, were concerned about being criticized because of language difficulties (in a multicultural classroom), or were worried about the quality of their work.

> Some students, for example, were concerned that a project they posted on the Padlet might not be good enough. This generated feelings of doubt about their work and stimulated thoughts that "maybe yours is less good than what the others did".

Assessment for Learning

The students reported that despite their concerns about collaboration, they were very quickly exposed to a variety of projects. The possibility of revising their projects based on comparisons with other projects or their classmates' assessment had a positive influence on their learning and on the learning product, enabling them to relate to new ideas and other perspectives.

> Seeing the projects of the other groups and being able to respond to and criticize what they did was something really excellent because [it] helped me understand what is desired and what is not. I was exposed to other presentation methods and other approaches to information. I felt that by reading the projects of other members of the group I accumulated new information. I learned how to condense material, how to critique someone who really worked hard and someone who may have done less, and how to criticize my own project and see how it can be improved. We even started asking other lecturers for permission to use the same method to complete their assignments.

Sharing projects and assignments enabled the students to assess their own work and that of their peers. As a result, they were able to revise their own projects. Thus they were exposed to a variety of ideas and perspectives as well as the implementation of diverse capabilities, such as self-criticism, comparison and synthesis of materials.

In final projects, students usually do not have the possibility of comparison with other students' projects. Frontal teaching often offers opportunities for discussing and comparing projects, whereas this may be problematic in a-synchronic or online learning formats. The students reported in their journals that the Padlet platform offered this possibility online, thus boosting their confidence, enriching their knowledge, and encouraging them toward higher-order thinking in the form of critiques and self-examination.

> Padlet helped me form additional opinions of the project I submitted. This would not have been the case had I sent the project directly to the lecturer on the website such that only the lecturer could see it. This gave me insight into the opinions of other students and showed me what things needed improvement.

Active Online Learning and Student Engagement

Another category emerging from analysis of the students' reflective journals concerns active learning and active engagement of students throughout the course, using the

Padlet digital platform. This categorical analysis revealed that the students found themselves actively involved in the learning processes and even experienced the active engagement of other students.

> It was amazing to see the responses of the students, and even more so when I was able to respond to the responses and questions of others regarding our assignment. The input from other students made me realize I had grown as a person and not only in terms of learning. I realized I have something to say and am able to think critically.

The students also noted that the option to add comments and communicate about the material facilitated brainstorming and discussion in writing, often over time. This brainstorming promoted open discussion. As a result, they were able to edit the material, construct arguments, and ground their arguments in the material studied, both individually and anonymously.

> I started responding to people. I expressed my opinion to others. I commented on topics that others raised on the Padlet. I liked very much how I responded to others and I enjoyed seeing that others responded to what I posted on the Padlet. In the end, my experience using Padlet gave me the possibility of examining various perspectives.

Difficulties and Limitations of the Platform

The students also reported difficulties in using this methodology, primarily in the initial stages when they were not familiar with it and sometimes needed to acquire additional information on their own about how to use the platform. The analysis revealed that even this experience of having to cope with a new situation ultimately made it easier for them to cope and was not accompanied by feelings of frustration.

> During the course of the project as we gained experience with the new technology (Padlet), we encountered several problems and difficulties in uploading the project and the text. At first we were unable to record [or] to connect all the recordings, and in addition it took us some time to understand how the Padlet works and responds and how to upload the assignment.
>
> At first, I had a hard time adjusting to the Padlet and I was a little worried about using it, but after I was exposed to using it I understood the importance of various learning technologies and constant developments in academia.

In this case as well, the students who reported initial problems in adjusting to the new methodology and unfamiliar technology reported that they were helped by other group members.

> At first, we found it a bit hard to get used to this new way of learning. And to tell you the truth, we did not manage to submit the project properly in real time, and the article didn't open for us in Padlet. Afterwards, another student helped us and sent us a link in the comment that did work.

> Padlet itself was technologically accessible and convenient and also, we always did the projects in groups so there was always someone who understood and could help.

Adaptation to New Technologies

During the activity, the students were given the opportunity to examine the platform and their work with other technologies. Indeed, they were given extensive guidance regarding the nature and form of the final project to enable them to make use of additional tools. Adopting technological tools is in itself a process of reinforcement. Indeed, as the students reported, their positive experience using Padlet removed barriers and concerns:

> After trying various learning technologies once or twice, I am no longer afraid of trying another new learning technology because I have already experienced several different technologies. This gives me a feeling of calm in that I know I will easily be able to cope and understand how to behave in new and unfamiliar situations.

Some of the students even noted that they gained more confidence in their ability to cope with changes and new situations that require adaptation to new learning technologies.

> My success in using Padlet increased my confidence. I derived great satisfaction from acquiring the new tool and from being able to implement this type of knowledge and learning.

> I learned something about myself: I learned that learning and research with the help of technological tools suits me. Indeed, even if it takes time to get used to and learn how to use a tool like this, the effort is worthwhile because technological tools make it easy and simple to gather information, articles, and studies on any required subject.

Cognitive Flexibility and High Order Thinking

Another category that derives from the proposed theory concerns cognitive flexibility and high-order thinking skills that emerged and developed in the students during the course of the intervention. The students reported that they had become aware of interaction and solution alternatives, began considering different opinions while interacting with their classmates, and were open to embracing new perspectives targeted at achieving better results. They indicated that collaborative learning enabled them to experience learning processes such as brainstorming, group discussion, disagreement resolution, and the exchange of ideas.

> I agreed with some of the opinions. Some amazed me because they were points I hadn't thought about or paid attention to before. Exposure to these ideas helped me formulate my own opinions and make my own choices.

Similarly, the students were exposed to diverse perspectives and contrary opinions. During the group discussions of the assignments they were able to experience stepping into someone else's shoes. This was also the case when they presented their final projects, which entailed receiving and writing critiques.

> This course required me to take an article and apply it to the organization we were dealing with, without remaining within a particular intellectual square or cube. Rather, I had to give

> myself the intellectual space for other topics and criticism and for deciphering the various topics. This requirement gave the project added value.

The fact that the projects were displayed visually on the board generated a competition of sorts for the attention of the viewer and the members of the other groups. This created a situation in which the students felt they had to improve their projects and be more precise in order to attract many responses and achieve high exposure. The students reported that they had to invest a great deal of time and effort in condensing the material and organizing it before they presented it. The stage of thinking about and processing the products of higher-order learning requires a high level of understanding, synthesis, selection, and written expression.

> The main difficulty I encountered throughout the course was that working with Padlet required being able to know how to condense the entire project into a few focal points and relevant sentences and to learn to choose what to put in the Padlet and what is less important to include in the main points.

> Because we wanted the other students in the course to want to read our project, we understood that we had to attract their attention. Therefore, we inserted a video clip at the opening of the Padlet in an attempt to condense the project as much as possible and to include only the important points... Doing this required a lot of discussion and collaborative thinking

As the semester progressed and the students became more proficient in using Padlet, they reported that they had honed these higher-order abilities and were able to cope with the ensuing assignments with fewer difficulties. They noted that these abilities continued to improve as they used the platform and as they compared their use and received help from other group members or members of other groups.

> The main difficulty was "condensing" a long text into "main points." This part required us to know which parts to relinquish and which parts to focus on... In our view, at first all the material seemed important. Only through experience were we able to view the text critically in order to devise an interesting and intriguing Padlet rather than one that was long and exhausting. But the benefit of this difficulty was that I learned to develop my ability to summarize and to establish priorities in presenting information. In the first assignment I did with the group members I felt I didn't contribute much in this regard, but in the final project I already felt more experienced.

Discussion

In this chapter, we delved into the implementation of the Padlet-mediated Online Collaborative Learning (OCL) methodology within health management education, showcasing how the Padlet platform can effectively facilitate this process. The analysis of health management students' reflective journals revealed a user-friendly experience with Padlet. This aligns with the expanded understanding of "user experience" that now encompasses design, information presentation, and emotional aspects, as well as the interface between technology and the individual (Minichiello et al., 2018). This positive user experience was crucial in motivating the students to actively use the platform, resembling their interactions on familiar social media platforms.

The Padlet platform proved essential in fostering social and learning interactions among health management students. It created an environment conducive to collaborative learning, exposing students to a diversity of viewpoints and enhancing their capacity for flexible decision-making in a healthcare context. This approach is supported by Cole et al. (2021), who highlighted the significance of students' perceptions of online learning environments in determining their engagement.

The participants reported a marked increase in activity levels, including the involvement of students from various backgrounds. Assignments were structured to facilitate the accumulation of shared knowledge, which was critical for the students' learning process. The user-friendly nature of Padlet contributed significantly to the success of this collaborative approach, fostering a sense of community, shared objectives, and a collaborative spirit essential in healthcare management.

The transition from individual to collaborative learning was initially challenging for students, often accompanied by anxiety over sharing work and fear of criticism. However, they gradually recognized the value of collaboration for professional growth, mirroring the dynamics in a healthcare setting where teamwork and interprofessional collaboration are key. This experience is reflective of the findings by Aldholay et al. (2018) regarding the promotion of higher-order outcomes through OCL.

For health management students, the benefits of using Padlet in large classes were particularly significant. It facilitated high levels of engagement and interaction, addressing the challenges of effectively teaching large groups in the contemporary educational landscape, as noted by Young and Nichols (2017). Padlet's ability to support highly engaged participation (Mehta et al., 2021) presents an effective solution for the challenges of modern healthcare education.

The students' engagement with the Padlet platform and the online methodology enhanced their cognitive flexibility and higher-order thinking, crucial for health professionals who must navigate complex, multifaceted environments. They learned to appreciate diverse perspectives, engage in critical discussions, and adapt to feedback—skills imperative in the health management sector. This development of cognitive flexibility and open-mindedness is aligned with the need for healthcare professionals to be adaptable, innovative, and responsive in their practice (Barak & Levenberg, 2016; Boot et al., 2017).

The evolving digital era, especially highlighted during the COVID-19 pandemic, has underscored the need for innovative teaching methods that promote active learning and engagement, particularly in health management education. These methods are vital for preparing health management professionals to effectively address the challenges and changes in the healthcare sector. Therefore, the focus on innovative teaching and learning technologies is not only a necessity but a critical component in the development of future health professionals, equipping them with the skills to thrive in a dynamic healthcare landscape.

References

Aldholay, A. H., Isaac, O., Abdullah, Z., & Ramayah, T. (2018). The role of transformational leadership as a mediating variable in DeLone and McLean information system success model: The context of online learning usage in Yemen. *Telematics and Informatics, 35*(5), 1421–1437. https://doi.org/10.1016/j.tele.2018.03.012

Alt, D., Raichel, N., & Naamati-Schneider, L. (2022). Higher education students' reflective journal writing and lifelong learning skills: Insights from an exploratory sequential study. *Frontiers in Psychology*. https://doi.org/10.3389/fpsyg.2021.707168

Balouchi, S., & Samad, A. A. (2021). No more excuses, learn English for free: Factors affecting L2 learners intention to use online technology for informal English learning. *Education and Information Technologies, 26*(1), 1111–1132. https://doi.org/10.1007/s10639-020-10307-z

Barak, M., & Levenberg, A. (2016). Flexible thinking in learning: An individual differences measure for learning in technology-enhanced environments. *Computers and Education, 99*, 39–52. https://doi.org/10.1016/j.compedu.2016.04.003

Beltrán-Martín, I. (2019). Using Padlet for collaborative learning. In *Proceedings HEAD'19. 5th International Conference on Higher Education Advances* (pp. 201–211). Editorial Universitat Politècnica de València.

Blieck, Y., Ooghe, I., Zhu, C., Depryck, K., Struyven, K., Pynoo, B., & Van Laer, H. (2019). Consensus among stakeholders about success factors and indicators for quality of online and blended learning in adult education: A Delphi study. *Studies in Continuing Education, 41*(1), 36–60.

Boot, N., Baas, M., van Gaal, S., Cools, R., & De Dreu, C. K. (2017). Creative cognition and dopaminergic modulation of fronto-striatal networks: Integrative review and research agenda. *Neuroscience and Biobehavioral Reviews, 78*, 13–23.

Cole, A. W., Lennon, L., & Weber, N. L. (2021). Student perceptions of online active learning practices and online learning climate predict online course engagement. *Interactive Learning Environments, 29*(5), 866–880. https://doi.org/10.1080/10494820.2019.1619593

DiPasquale, J. (2017). Wiki'd transgressions: Scaffolding still necessary to support online collaborative learning. *Canadian Journal of Action Research, 18*(3), 47–61. https://doi.org/10.33524/cjar.v18i3.355

Gasmi, A. A., & Thomas, M. (2017). Academic writing in the flipped EFL classroom: A case study on student engagement in Oman. In *Flipped instruction methods and digital technologies in the language learning classroom* (pp. 232–251). IGI Global.

Grosser, J., Bientzle, M., & Kimmerle, J. (2020). A literature review on the foundations and potentials of digital teaching scenarios for interprofessional health care education. *International Journal of Environmental Research and Public Health, 17*(10), 3410. https://doi.org/10.3390/ijerph17103410

Männistö, M., Mikkonen, K., Kuivila, H. M., Virtanen, M., Kyngäs, H., & Kääriäinen, M. (2020). Digital collaborative learning in nursing education: A systematic review. *Scandinavian Journal of Caring Sciences, 34*(2), 280–292.

Mehta K. J., Miletich I., & Detyna M. (2021). Content-specific differences in Padlet perception for collaborative learning amongst undergraduate students. *Research in Learning Technology, 29*. https://doi.org/10.25304/rlt.v29.2551

Minichiello, A., Hood, J. R., & Harkness, D. S. (2018). Bringing user experience design to bear on STEM education: A narrative literature review. *Journal for STEM Education Research, 1*, 7–33. https://doi.org/10.1007/s41979-018-0005-3

Naamati-Schneider, L., & Alt, D. (2023a). Online collaborative Padlet-mediated learning in health management studies. *Frontiers in Psychology, 14*, 1157621. https://doi.org/10.3389/fpsyg.2023.1157621

Naamati-Schneider, L., & Alt, D. (2023b). Enhancing collaborative learning in health management education: An investigation of Padlet-mediated interventions and the influence of flexible thinking. *BMC Medical Education, 23*(1), 846. https://doi.org/10.1186/s12909-023-04796-y

Ng, P. M., Chan, J. K., & Lit, K. K. (2022). Student learning performance in online collaborative learning. *Education and Information Technologies, 27*(6), 8129–8145. https://doi.org/10.1007/s10639-022-10923-x

Park, C. W., Kim, D. G., Cho, S., & Han, H. J. (2019). Adoption of multimedia technology for learning and gender difference. *Computers in Human Behavior, 92*, 288–296. https://doi.org/10.1016/j.chb.2018.11.029

Qureshi, M. A., Khaskheli, A., Qureshi, J. A., Raza, S. A., & Yousufi, S. Q. (2023). Factors affecting students' learning performance through collaborative learning and engagement. *Interactive Learning Environments, 31*(4), 2371–2391. https://doi.org/10.1080/10494820.2021.1884886

Rashid, A. A., Yunus, M. M., & Wahi, W. (2019). Using Padlet for collaborative writing among ESL learners. *Creative Education, 10*(3), 610–620. https://doi.org/10.4236/ce.2019.103044

Sukendro, S., Habibi, A., Khaeruddin, K., Indrayana, B., Syahruddin, S., Makadada, F. A., & Hakim, H. (2020). Using an extended technology acceptance model to understand students' use of e-learning during Covid-19: Indonesian sport science education context. *Heliyon, 6*(11), e05410.https://doi.org/10.1016/j.heliyon.2020.e05410

Yadegaridehkordi, E., Shuib, L., Nilashi, M., & Asadi, S. (2019). Decision to adopt online collaborative learning tools in higher education: A case of top Malaysian universities. *Education and Information Technologies, 24*(1), 79–102. https://doi.org/10.1007/s10639-018-9761-z

Young, S., & Nichols, H. (2017). A reflexive evaluation of technology-enhanced learning. *Research in Learning Technology, 25*. https://doi.org/10.25304/rlt.v25.1998

Zheng, L., Chen, N. S., Huang, R., & Yang, K. (2014). A novel approach to assess collaborative learning processes and group performance through the knowledge convergence. *Journal of Computers in Education, 1*, 167–185. https://doi.org/10.1007/s40692-014-0009-7

Chapter 12
Integrating AI into Healthcare: Implications for Medical Education and Management

Abstract Leveraging the transformative potential of AI in healthcare administration and medical care is essential for future advancements. This chapter explores the impact of AI tools at all system levels, addressing implementation challenges. It emphasizes integrating AI into education and training programs in higher education and medical institutions, highlighting the need for new competencies among healthcare managers and professionals. The chapter reviews innovative initiatives embedding these competencies in academic and organizational contexts, preparing a forward-thinking workforce for future challenges.

Introduction

In recent years, the local and global healthcare environment has faced increasing changes, which further accelerated in December 2019, in the wake of the COVID outbreak. Given these changes, health systems must take concrete steps to help health professionals acquire new skills to facilitate adaptation to change at all levels (Deshpande et al., 2023; Naamati-Schneider, 2020, 2022). Over the past decade, as healthcare organizations sought to adapt to this changing environment, they began to embrace the notion of generating change through digital transformation and digital tools. This direction has served a variety of goals, such as enhancing organizational performance, improving customer care, streamlining organizational processes, gaining a competitive advantage and implementing innovative business models (Naamati-Schneider, 2020; Naamati-Schneider & Salvatore, 2022, 2023). Among these digital tools, artificial intelligence (AI) tools have begun to be implemented both in business management and in medical care (Ali et al., 2023; Jimma, 2023; Manne & Kantheti, 2021; Younis et al., 2024).

AI is defined as the use of computer systems to perform tasks that typically require human intelligence, such as visual perception, speech recognition, decision-making, and language translation. AI systems can learn from data, identify patterns, and make predictions or recommendations based on that data. AI technologies aim to mimic human cognitive functions through technological means, particularly machine

L. Naamati-Schneider and D. Alt, *Technology and Competency-Oriented Learning*,
https://doi.org/10.1007/978-981-97-5771-8_12

learning. This approach makes it easier to analyze data, draw conclusions and make accurate predictions. Indeed, the ability to process massive amounts of information in real time constitutes a significant advantage over the human ability to process data. Hence, AI may be applied regularly in different arenas and domains for individuals, organizations, and even large governmental systems and countries (Aiello, 2024; Aronson, 2022; Jiang et al., 2017; Mikalef et al., 2022; Tekkeşin, 2019).

AI has both significant advantages and potential drawbacks. Indeed, as this technology has advanced and become more accessible, the complexities surrounding its use in various industries have begun to emerge. Awareness is growing in both the public and academic spheres of the need to regulate and manage the potential risks posed by this technology. These risks include threats posed to various social sectors, such as the labor market, professional fields, educational systems, legal rights and regulations, and even the future of humanity as a whole (Aiello, 2024; Ali et al., 2023; Manne & Kantheti, 2021; Olorunsogo et al., 2024).

Yet undoubtedly AI also offers many benefits. The advancement of artificial intelligence has generated remarkable power and efficacy across multiple domains, particularly in healthcare and medical services. Integrating AI into the medical sector has vast and promising potential, offering opportunities to enhance both treatment and service management. AI is increasingly being used in healthcare to improve disease diagnosis, treatment, and outcome prediction (Jiang et al., 2017; Jimma, 2023; Naamati-Schneider, 2023; Rahman et al., 2024; Younis et al., 2024).

To fully harness the benefits of AI technology while minimizing its risks, significant time and resources must be invested in planning and regulating its use. This requires conducting a great deal of research in this area. As of now, the scarcity of relevant research has resulted in a significant information and knowledge deficit regarding the impact of employing these tools in educational and work-based environments. Expanded knowledge together with planning and regulation will enable systems, organizations and individuals at various levels to accommodate and adapt to the expected changes (Ali et al., 2023; Manne & Kantheti, 2021).

This chapter explores the potential applications of AI tools in medical administration and care across all levels of the healthcare system. It highlights the challenges and barriers of using AI in medical settings that must be addressed in preparation for this change. The discussion also focuses on the integration of AI tools in institutions of higher education and training programs that prepare people for the medical professions. It underscores the need to cultivate a novel set of competencies among healthcare managers and professionals to enable them to adapt to this new setting. These competencies will enable healthcare workers at all levels to accommodate and acclimate to the changes brought on by the use of AI in healthcare. In addition, the chapter surveys current creative initiatives aimed at implementing these capabilities in academic and organizational healthcare settings.

The Present and Future of AI Integration Across All Levels of Healthcare System

The healthcare sector is currently witnessing a significant shift towards incorporating AI technologies in different domains. In this section, we discuss the impact of AI implementation in healthcare at three levels: macro, meso, and micro. As noted throughout this book, these levels correspond to different domains of the healthcare system, ranging from broad holistic social structures to individual behavior.

According to a special report on the use of AI in healthcare published in 2020 by the National Academy of Medicine, the use of AI in healthcare shows a great deal of promise, offering many potential opportunities for improving patient outcomes, reducing costs, and exerting a positive impact on the health of the population (Matheny et al., 2020).

AI Macro-level Implications

The use of AI at the macro-level has many implications, among them system standardization, setting system guidelines, and planning and budgeting for acquiring, developing and assimilating new digital technologies and AI tools that will facilitate efficient, sustainable and high-quality treatment and service (Vyas et al., 2023).

Due to the significant risks and ethical challenges involved in AI use, the healthcare system and its key stakeholders must take regulatory steps at the macro level to ensure patient safety and promote responsible innovation. Implementing an overall system approach to address the clinical use of AI can create a context in which regulators can collaborate and support each other so that AI use can simultaneously meet multiple regulatory goals (TerKonda & Fish, 2023).

Moreover, to better address the challenges of using AI and to maximize its benefits, healthcare system managers must integrate educational planning and budgeting into the curricula of medical, nursing, and other health-related programs. AI must be included as part of the overall planning and standardization of professional skills in the field of health. Indeed, education can serve as a critical component in promoting responsible use of artificial intelligence in healthcare while ensuring patient safety (Chan, 2023; Fuchs, 2023; TerKonda & Fish, 2023; York et al., 2023; Zhang et al., 2024).

AI Meso-level Implications

The meso level of the healthcare system refers to the organizations and the intermediate levels at which actions are implemented and management strategies are formulated. Critical managerial and operational decisions related to budgeting, resourcing, operating procedures, and human resource management are all made at the meso level. Hence, integrating AI into clinical and administrative processes at this level will have a profound impact, as AI can significantly outperform humans in terms of accuracy, efficiency, and timely execution of medical and other related administrative processes (Ali et al., 2023; Manne & Kantheti, 2021; Naamati-Schneider, 2023).

AI technologies are already being used today to support clinical decision-making, diagnosis, and treatment. Machine learning algorithms can analyze patient data and offer valuable insights into disease patterns, thus helping doctors make informed decisions (Göndöcs & Dörfler, 2024). AI chatbots provide patients with ongoing support in the form of self-diagnosis and general health advice that is available around the clock. Additionally, medical devices powered by AI, such as wearable sensors, collect real-time data on patients' vital signs and transmit this information to healthcare providers for remote monitoring (Yu et al., 2018). AI is also used in remote care by monitoring patients remotely, reducing the need for frequent visits to healthcare providers (Rong et al., 2020).

AI is also used to enhance the quality of service delivery in the healthcare industry by providing personalized and efficient care. For example, AI-powered virtual assistants can help patients book appointments, find the nearest clinic, and be reminded when to take their medication. AI chatbots can also help patients navigate insurance requirements, reducing the administrative burden on healthcare providers. Moreover, AI chatbots can assist patients with filing insurance claims, thus reducing the administrative workload for healthcare providers (Ali et al., 2023). AI can also be used to automate repetitive administrative tasks, thus freeing healthcare providers to focus on delivering high-quality care to patients. AI can assist in organizing patient flow and reducing bureaucracy in healthcare systems and also improve management processes in the healthcare industry by analyzing vast amounts of data to identify patterns and trends. Predictive models powered by AI can forecast patient demand for specific services, enabling healthcare providers to allocate resources more efficiently. AI can also analyze patient feedback and suggest areas for improvement in service delivery. Moreover, AI models can be used to identify and predict the efficacy of potential new drugs, thus streamlining clinical trials and reducing both time and cost (Ali et al., 2024; Manne & Kantheti, 2021; Visan & Negut, 2024).

AI undoubtedly has the potential to revolutionize the healthcare industry and the performance of healthcare organizations by improving clinical decision-making, enhancing service quality, and optimizing management processes. Nevertheless, the extent to which healthcare organizations will adopt and use these tools in routine medical care in the near and far future will depend on their commitment to implementing innovative and complementary working methods and developing applications that will replace existing techniques, for example applications that analyze the results of medical tests, compare data, conduct genetic tests, perform necessary statistical calculations for diagnosis and prognosis, and more (Ali et al., 2023, 2024; Jiang et al., 2017).

AI Micro-level Implications

An organization's micro level refers to the individual level of the healthcare professionals (e.g., managers and medical staff) working in the organization. Integration of AI on this level will affect both patients and caregivers in multiple ways and will generate a shift in their relationship. Indeed, the patient-caregiver relationship has evolved over the past decade, from a paternalistic relationship to a more collaborative partnership. Today, as the role of caregivers changes and they begin to serve more as mediators than authorities in the field, this relationship is likely to change again. Indeed, with the advancement of AI technology, the role of the caregiver may become less essential, forcing healthcare professionals to adopt new notions regarding their roles, responsibility, and accountability (Figueroa et al., 2019; Kerstan et al., 2024). The aforementioned changes may result in blurred boundaries and accountability issues. As the roles and authority of the caregiver become unclear, there is a risk of reduced accountability, transparency, and understanding of individual responsibilities. This can create instability and potentially lead to medical and managerial problems (Longenecker & Longenecker, 2014). At the same time, AI can offer significant benefits to patients by improving diagnosis, treatment, consultation, and health monitoring for self-management of acute and chronic conditions (Sqalli & Al-Thani, 2019). AI can aid in early disease identification, optimize treatment plans, provide virtual consultations, and allow for remote health monitoring (Ali et al., 2023). AI can also be utilized in personalized medicine to develop individualized treatment plans based on a patient's distinct genetic profile and medical history, leading to customized treatment and a unique patient-caregiver relationship (Manne & Kantheti, 2021). Hence, the introduction of AI necessitates changes in the patient-caregiver relationship, as both sides are forced to adopt different work and behavior patterns (Allen et al., 2024; Ryan & Sysko, 2007).

Processes occurring at the micro level are also compelling healthcare professionals to adapt to major cultural, organizational, managerial, and personal changes. To this end, they must receive training in a range of skills and capabilities to prepare them to embrace change, be creative, innovative, and flexible, and be able to use AI tools effectively.

Challenges and Barriers in the Use of AI in Medical Settings

The incorporation of AI tools and technologies will undoubtedly bring enormous benefits to patients, healthcare professionals, administrators, and the entire healthcare organization and system. Nevertheless, like any innovative process, the use of AI in healthcare brings with it significant challenges, barriers and threats that need to be addressed (Li et al., 2024; Matheny et al., 2020; Sallam, 2023; York et al., 2023). These challenges can be categorized into three dimensions: data challenges, legal challenges and patient challenges.

The first dimension of data challenges encompasses data digitization and consolidation, data availability, and data integrity. Data challenges may serve as a barrier to the implementation of AI systems as they require high-quality processing and automation (Manne & Kantheti, 2021), as in the case of AI performance evaluation and the lack of standards for assessing the safety and efficacy of AI systems. The US FDA has made initial attempts to provide guidance for assessing AI systems, but further development is needed. Another example in this dimension is the challenge posed by data exchange. AI systems must be continuously trained with data from clinical studies, but the healthcare environment does not provide incentives for sharing data within the system (Jiang et al., 2017).

The second dimension of legal challenges entails privacy and security issues, ethical issues, and government regulations (Jimma, 2023; Morley & Floridi, 2019). The challenges presented by privacy/legal issues are a concern for healthcare organizations due to the confidentiality and complexity of medical data. The use of AI in healthcare involves collecting, processing, and storing sensitive patient data, raising concerns about data privacy and security. Indeed, if patients are not confident that their data will be kept confidential and secure they may be hesitant to share their private health information with healthcare providers (Ali et al., 2023). Furthermore, AI algorithms are designed to make decisions based on data, but these decisions can have significant consequences for patients. The risk is that AI algorithms may make decisions that are not in patients' best interest or that may be biased against certain groups of patients. This risk raises ethical concerns about the use of AI in healthcare, pointing to the need for clear guidelines and regulations to ensure that AI is used in an ethical and responsible manner that respects patients' privacy and autonomy. For this reason, ethical principles such as transparency, accountability and fairness must be incorporated into the development and deployment of AI systems in healthcare (Morley & Floridi, 2019).

The third dimension of patient challenges includes decision errors, treatment errors, data errors, and human interventions, all of which may compromise patient safety. One of the main risks is of potential harm to patients if the AI tools are not properly designed, tested, and regulated. There is also a risk that AI use may lead to a reduction in quality of care, particularly if physicians become overly reliant on the technology and fail to exercise and trust their own clinical judgment. Additionally, the use of AI runs the risk of exacerbating existing health disparities if the algorithms are not designed to account for different patient populations (TerKonda & Fish, 2023).

A study by Manne and Kantheti (2021) demonstrated further challenges and barriers to the use of AI in medical settings. The study examined the implications and challenges for healthcare management of using AI in healthcare settings. One challenge involves the need for a large amount of data to train AI models effectively. In healthcare, obtaining large amounts of data can be difficult due to privacy concerns and the individual variability of diseases. Additionally, because healthcare data are often ambiguous, noisy, and incomplete, applying AI in healthcare is more challenging than in other fields. Another challenge is that clinicians are slow to adopt technological changes. Healthcare workers need to be trained to use AI applications effectively, and the applications themselves must be user-friendly to encourage their adoption.

The challenges outlined above may act as barriers to the adoption and improvement of AI practices in healthcare and may serve as valid reasons for organizations and employees to resist adopting and safely using AI tools. Nevertheless, despite concerns that the potential risks will stop or restrict the use of these tools, their adoption is likely to continue to accelerate and become more widespread in the future. Therefore, curricula and training programs in higher education institutions and professional medical and management training must be adapted to encourage responsible and safe use of these tools (Matheny et al., 2020). Furthermore, medical training programs must strive to build and implement a set of competencies that facilitate the optimal use of these tools and minimize resistance while ensuring their safe use over time. Educators must seek to integrate AI tools into educational curricula and to develop the necessary skills to match their use, thus enhancing their functionality and improving the learning experience.

The next section focuses on integrating AI tools into educational programs and developing the skills medical personnel need to be able to use AI, thus increasing the effectiveness of these tools and optimizing learning outcomes.

Integrating AI in Education: Teaching with and Using AI

Education plays a crucial role in promoting the responsible use of artificial intelligence in healthcare while ensuring patient safety. Indeed, educators must ensure that healthcare professionals have the necessary clinical and ethical competence to use algorithm-based treatments and to explain to patients the reasoning behind their diagnoses and treatments (Eysenbach, 2023; TerKonda & Fish, 2023; Zhang et al., 2024).

In order to ensure and develop the ability of healthcare professionals to use diverse AI tools and integrate them into their daily professional work, these tools must be taught at the early stages of learning, e.g., to undergraduate students or those in their first year of professional training. By experimenting with these tools, users can improve their skills and gain confidence in their own abilities, while at the same time becoming more familiar with the tools' limitations (Ali et al., 2023; Eysenbach, 2023; York et al., 2023). This is exemplified by a study conducted by York et al. (2023), which sought to investigate how doctors and medical students perceived the use of AI technology in skeletal radiology. The study examined participants' pre-existing knowledge of AI, their confidence in interpreting plain radiographs for skeletal trauma, and their projected confidence in using an AI system to identify positive and negative X-rays. The study found that the majority of participants held a generally favorable view of AI technology in healthcare and believed that it would be beneficial. Yet the study also revealed a generally low knowledge of AI among the participants, indicating that medical curricula needed to provide additional training in AI use.

In addition, innovative AI tools can also be beneficial in teaching itself. These tools can enhance knowledge of different teaching and learning methods and maximize holistic use of time and technology for effective and high-quality learning. By promoting awareness and ethical discussions about the implications and challenges of AI tools, healthcare educators can establish a regulatory framework for learners and professional users of AI, thus reducing the risks and barriers to AI use.

The incorporation of Artificial Intelligence-based Language Learning Models (LLMs) such as ChatGTP is an example of using AI in teaching. ChatGTP is a set of AI-powered applications that use natural language processing and machine learning algorithms to understand and generate human-like language. The applications can be used to generate text, answer questions, and engage in conversations with humans. In the context of healthcare education, AI-based LLMs such as ChatGPT can be used to provide personalized and interactive learning experiences for students, as well as to simplify complex medical concepts. To this end, ChatGPT can generate tailored responses to student queries, recommend relevant learning resources, and adapt content to individual learning needs. For example, ChatGPT can generate personalized quiz questions based on the learning progress of individual students, recommend additional resources based on students' knowledge gaps, and adapt explanations to match their preferred learning style. Furthermore, ChatGPT can simplify complex medical concepts by generating natural language explanations, simplifying medical jargon into layman's terms, providing additional examples or analogies to clarify difficult concepts, and suggesting links to relevant resources to deepen students' understanding (Sallam 2023).

ChatGPT can also help in generating effective patient discharge summaries and providing easily accessible and understandable health information to learners. ChatGPT can be used for automated scoring and providing teaching assistance, for example by generating exercises and quizzes and creating virtual tutors to provide personalized learning. It can also be used for research assistance by providing quick access to information, generating case scenarios for medical students, creating content for learning, and offering language translation for medical professionals.

Nevertheless, the use of ChatGPT in healthcare education is also associated with various risks and concerns, among them ethical, transparency, and legal issues, as well as risks associated with bias, plagiarism, inaccurate content, limited knowledge, incorrect citations, cybersecurity issues, and infodemics. For these reasons, ChatGPT should not be seen as a replacement for human teachers and educators (Khan et al., 2023; Sallam, 2023).

The work of Eysenbach (2023) illustrates the importance of guidance and regulation in the use of AI. In a series of conversations with Chat GTP, Eysenbach suggested a number of ideas regarding how the tool can be integrated into medical studies. In response, ChatGTP generated many good options, among them essay grading and feedback, creating virtual patients for medical training, enhancing medical textbooks by generating additional explanations, examples, and visual aids, summarizing medical research articles, and highlighting the key findings and implications of a study. Nevertheless, ChatGTP may also generate incorrect responses or invented data (e.g., references), leading to student error and misinformation when students lack critical thinking skills.

Han et al. (2023) similarly examined the use of ChatGPT as a potential tool for medical education by prompting the chatbot with learning objectives and tasks. The researchers found that while ChatGPT was able to provide basic information and explanations, it also had limitations and sometimes provided incorrect or incomplete information. The article emphasized the importance of active learning and critical thinking in medical education and the need for students to develop a deeper understanding of the basic sciences and their relevance to clinical medicine. The authors also pointed out that expert supervision and care are needed to ensure that the information generated is accurate and useful to students.

Das et al. (2023) also examined an attempt to integrate and assess ChatGPT's ability to answer first- and second-order knowledge questions related to microbiology and to determine its potential as an automated question-answering system for medical students. The result indicated that ChatGPT was able to answer first- and second-order knowledge questions related to microbiology with approximately 80% accuracy, indicating its potential as an automated question-answering system for medical students. Yet the researchers also noted that ongoing improvement in the training and development of language models is necessary to enhance their performance and make them suitable for academic use.

Likewise, researchers in the field of dental education (Das et al., 2023; Thurzo et al., 2023) have called for more research in the field AI education. According to them, the rapid development of AI technology and its impact on dentistry necessitates an update to dental curricula. They claimed that the use of AI in dentistry will lead to placing more emphasis on technology and data analytics in dental education. Consequently, dental professionals will need to master these tools to provide the best possible care to their patients. Hence, dental education undoubtedly must adapt to these changes to ensure that dental professionals are prepared to use AI in their practice. As is the case for other healthcare professionals, the results for dental professionals highlight the fact that AI implementation must be carefully managed to ensure that its benefits are realized while minimizing potential risks.

Recent digital advancements, particularly in AI tools, have increased access to digital information, emphasizing the need for medical professionals to develop skills for processing and verifying this information (Hemmo-Lotem & Shani, 2018; Schwab, 2017; Veikkolainen et al., 2023). Among these, digital health literacy skills are crucial. However, with the emergence of AI and language models like ChatGPT, the scope of digital literacy is transforming. It now requires not only traditional digital skills for searching and synthesizing information but also skills in understanding and working with AI. While the need for conventional digital skills may decrease as AI systems become more user-friendly, critical evaluation skills remain vital due to current limitations in AI credibility. Understanding context, recognizing biases, critically evaluating information, and making ethical judgments are areas where AI is still developing. These traditional digital skills, although potentially less relied upon over time, are significant in today's evolving AI landscape. Additionally, the rise of language models necessitates developing effective prompting skills (Eager & Brunton, 2023; Kasneci et al., 2023).

Recent research has highlighted the transformative impact of AI-powered assistants like ChatGPT on digital literacy skills within educational settings. A study by Naamati-Schneider and Alt (2024) compared traditional problem-based learning (PBL) and lecture-based learning (LBL) with AI-integrated problem-based learning (AIPBL) in healthcare management students. This comparison revealed that while PBL improves all three components of digital literacy—access, analysis, and evaluation—AIPBL specifically enhances evaluation skills but does not significantly impact access and analysis skills. This suggests that while AI tools can reshape educational methodologies and student competencies, they also necessitate a reevaluation of the skills deemed essential for contemporary digital literacy. The integration of AI into educational systems emphasizes the evolving role of traditional literacy skills and the emerging necessity for advanced AI literacy skills to navigate the digital landscape effectively.

In the realm of healthcare management, proficiency in digital literacy and AI-related skills has transitioned from a beneficial asset to an essential requirement. Healthcare managers utilizing AI tools can significantly enhance strategic decision-making and operational efficiency through several means. Firstly, AI enables data-driven decision-making, allowing managers to base their strategies on comprehensive data analyses, such as patient outcomes and resource utilization. Predictive analytics provided by AI aids in forecasting healthcare trends, from patient admissions to potential disease outbreaks, facilitating more effective planning and resource allocation. Personalized healthcare management is another frontier where AI's capabilities can be harnessed, enabling managers to oversee individualized patient care strategies, thereby improving patient outcomes and satisfaction. In terms of operational efficiency, AI optimizes various aspects of hospital management, including staff scheduling and inventory management, leading to cost reductions and improved service delivery. Additionally, AI tools are instrumental in ensuring quality control and compliance with healthcare standards and regulations. They also play a critical role in risk management by identifying potential safety concerns or inefficiencies. Beyond these practical applications, AI enhances communication and coordination within healthcare facilities, streamlining workflows and fostering teamwork. Importantly, healthcare managers must navigate the ethical dimensions of AI use, particularly regarding patient privacy and algorithmic bias, ensuring responsible and ethical decision-making. Finally, the rapid evolution of AI technology necessitates a commitment to continual learning and adaptation among healthcare managers, ensuring that they remain at the forefront of leveraging advanced tools for the betterment of healthcare delivery and administration. This comprehensive integration of AI skills underscores their criticality in contemporary healthcare management.

Discussion

Artificial intelligence is predicted to be the next revolutionary technology that will transform the world as we know it. We are still in the early stages of embracing AI and fully learning about its capabilities. Nevertheless, it is clear that AI will play a significant role in shaping our future. Incorporating AI in the world of healthcare and adapting to the resulting digital transformations will be crucial. Indeed, the implementation of AI technologies poses significant challenges and raises a number of questions to which there are still no clear answers.

At the time of writing this chapter, the future extent of these changes remains unclear, as does how they will affect all areas and levels of the health system and its workforce. What is clear is that we must prepare by teaching individuals and organizations to adapt to this changing environment. The challenges associated with the use of AI in healthcare include concerns regarding patient privacy; ethical, legal, and medical challenges related to the use of AI in making decisions about human lives and medical conditions; and potential harm to patients caused by system errors. These challenges need to be addressed to ensure that AI is used in a safe, effective, and ethical manner in healthcare.

Creating a supportive ethical and legal regulatory framework that upholds ethical and egalitarian principles is becoming increasingly important for the use of AI in the present and the future. Such a framework must include regulation of processes for developing and using these tools to emphasize their limitations and risks, while attempting to reduce errors and misuse. Standards should be established for using AI for learning or training, thus creating a safe experiential framework for the use of AI tools and the development of a skill set adapted to meet future demands. AI has the potential to transform healthcare services and improve the quality of care. Nevertheless, AI must be used responsibly to ensure its safe and effective use in healthcare (Jimma, 2023; Olorunsogo et al., 2024).

Caution must be taken to regulate the use of Artificial Intelligence-based Language Learning Models such as ChatGPT and similar tools in health education. To this end, ethical guidelines for use must be developed that incorporate human oversight and feedback, regularly monitor for potential errors or bias, and ensure compliance with relevant privacy regulations and policies. In this way, we can ensure that ChatGPT and other AI-based LLMs are used in a responsible and ethical manner, maximizing their potential benefits while minimizing their risks (Sallam, 2023). In this context, academic institutions must adopt learning methods and strategies suitable for online environments. Furthermore, instructors need to be trained on how to effectively incorporate AI into their classes. The same way, medical management and healthcare education institutions should actively integrate AI tools, including language models like ChatGPT, into their curricula to leverage their varied benefits. This integration not only exposes students to advanced technologies but also enhances their skills, particularly in effective AI tool usage like prompting (Naamati-Schneider, 2024; Naamati-Schneider & Alt, 2024). Mastering prompting skills is essential as it enables individuals to effectively communicate with and guide AI systems, ensuring more accurate, relevant, and useful responses from the technology. Simultaneously, it's vital to nurture critical thinking and evaluation abilities. These skills are key for students to competently navigate AI's limitations and challenges. Educators play a crucial role in guiding students to critically analyze AI-generated information, recognize biases, and employ AI responsibly, thus ensuring a balanced use of technology in educational settings. They must recognize the role of the teacher as a facilitator of learning while striving to design successful scaffolding strategies to develop students' knowledge and skills in prompting, computational thinking, up to date digital literacy, ethical judgment, critical thinking and as part of lifelong learning skills essential in today's world.

Furthermore, researchers must continue to examine and extend existing knowledge about the ramifications of implementing AI tools in different arenas while addressing potential shortcomings and ethical concerns (Manne & Kantheti, 2021; Sallam, 2023).

References

Aiello, M. (2024). The AI revolution and the future of work: Threats and opportunities. *Computer, 57*(05), 29–34. https://doi.ieeecomputersociety.org/10.1109/MC.2024.3374279

Ali, O., Abdelbaki, W., Shrestha, A., Elbasi, E., Alryalat, M. A. A., & Dwivedi, Y. K. (2023). A systematic literature review of artificial intelligence in the healthcare sector: Benefits, challenges, methodologies, and functionalities. *Journal of Innovation and Knowledge, 8*(1), 100333. https://doi.org/10.1016/j.jik.2023.100333

Ali, K. A., Mohin, S. K., Mondal, P., Goswami, S., Ghosh, S., & Choudhuri, S. (2024). Influence of artificial intelligence in modern pharmaceutical formulation and drug development. *Future Journal of Pharmaceutical Sciences, 10*(1), 53. https://doi-org.mgs.hac.ac.il/10.1186/s43094-024-00625-1

Allen, M. R., Webb, S., Mandvi, A., Frieden, M., Tai-Seale, M., & Kallenberg, G. (2024). Navigating the doctor-patient-AI relationship-a mixed-methods study of physician attitudes toward artificial intelligence in primary care. *BMC Primary Care, 25*(1), 42. https://doi-org.mgs.hac.ac.il/10.1186/s12875-024-02282-y

Aronson, J. K. (2022). Artificial intelligence in pharmacovigilance: An introduction to terms, concepts, applications, and limitations. *Drug Safety, 45*(5), 407–418. https://doi.org/10.1007/s40264-022-01156-5

Chan, C. K. Y. (2023). A comprehensive AI policy education framework for university teaching and learning. *International Journal of Educational Technology in Higher Education, 20*(1), 1–25. https://doi.org/10.1186/s41239-023-00408-3

Das, D., Kumar, N., Longjam, L. A., Sinha, R., Roy, A. D., Mondal, H., & Gupta, P. (2023). Assessing the capability of ChatGPT in answering first-and second-order knowledge questions on microbiology as per competency-based medical education curriculum. *Cureus, 15*(3). https://doi.org/10.7759/cureus.36034

Deshpande, N., Arora, V. M., Vollbrecht, H., Meltzer, D. O., & Press, V. (2023). EHealth literacy and patient portal use and attitudes: Cross-sectional observational study. *JMIR Human Factors, 10*, e40105. https://doi.org/10.2196/40105

Eager, B., & Brunton, R. (2023). Prompting higher education towards AI-augmented teaching and learning practice. *Journal of University Teaching and Learning Practice, 20*(5). https://doi.org/10.53761/1.20.5.02

Eysenbach, G. (2023). The role of ChatGPT, generative language models, and artificial intelligence in medical education: A conversation With ChatGPT and a call for papers. *JMIR Medical Education, 9*, e46885. https://doi.org/10.2196/46885

Figueroa, C. A., Harrison, R., Chauhan, A., & Meyer, L. (2019). Priorities and challenges for health leadership and workforce management globally: A rapid review. *BMC Health Services Research, 19*(1), 1–11. https://doi.org/10.1186/s12913-019-4080-7

Fuchs, K. (2023). Exploring the opportunities and challenges of NLP models in higher education: Is Chat GPT a blessing or a curse? *Frontiers in Education*. https://doi.org/10.3389/feduc.2023.1166682.8

Göndöcs, D., & Dörfler, V. (2024). AI in medical diagnosis: AI prediction and human judgment. *Artificial Intelligence in Medicine, 149*. https://doi.org/10.1016/j.artmed.2024.102769

Han, Z., Battaglia, F., Udaiyar, A., Fooks, A., & Terlecky, S. R. (2023). An explorative assessment of ChatGPT as an aid in medical education: Use it with caution. *medRxiv, 2*. https://doi.org/10.1101/2023.02.13.23285879

Hemmo-Lotem, M., & Shani, M. (2018). Changing the paradigm in medicine in the wake of the fourth industrial revolution. *Hrefuaa (The Medicine), 157*, 797–801. (Hebrew).

Jiang, F., Jiang, Y., Zhi, H., Dong, Y., Li, H., Ma, S., Wang, Y., Dong, Q., Shen, H., & Wang, Y. (2017). Artificial intelligence in healthcare: Past, present and future. *Stroke and Vascular Neurology, 2*(4), e000101. https://doi.org/10.1136/svn-2017-000101

Jimma, B. L. (2023). Artificial intelligence in healthcare: A bibliometric analysis. *Telematics and Informatics Reports*, 100041. https://doi.org/10.1016/j.teler.2023.100041

Kasneci, E., Seßler, K., Küchemann, S., Bannert, M., Dementieva, D., Fischer, F., Gasser, U., Groh, G., Günnemann, S., Hüllermeier, E., Krusche, S., & Kasneci, G. (2023). ChatGPT for good? On opportunities and challenges of large language models for education. *Learning and Individual Differences, 103*, 102274. https://doi.org/10.1016/j.lindif.2023.102274

Kerstan, S., Bienefeld, N., & Grote, G. (2024). Choosing human over AI doctors? How comparative trust associations and knowledge relate to risk and benefit perceptions of AI in healthcare. *Risk Analysis, 44*(4). https://doi-org.mgs.hac.ac.il/10.1111/risa.14216

Khan, R. A., Jawaid, M., Khan, A. R., & Sajjad, M. (2023). ChatGPT—Reshaping medical education and clinical management. *Pakistan Journal of Medical Sciences, 39*(2), 605–607. https://doi.org/10.12669/pjms.39.2.7653

Li, W., Ge, X., Liu, S., Xu, L., Zhai, X., & Yu, L. (2024). Opportunities and challenges of traditional Chinese medicine doctors in the era of artificial intelligence. *Frontiers in Medicine, 10* https://doi.org/10.3389/fmed.2023.1336175

Longenecker, C. O., & Longenecker, P. D. (2014). Why hospital improvement efforts fail: A view from the front line. *Journal of Healthcare Management, 59*(2), 147–157.

Manne, R., & Kantheti, S. C. (2021). Application of artificial intelligence in healthcare: Chances and challenges. *Current Journal of Applied Science and Technology, 40*(6), 78–89. https://doi.org/10.9734/cjast/2021/v40i631320

Matheny, M. E., Whicher, D., & Thadaney Israni, S. (2020). Artificial intelligence in health care: A report from the national academy of medicine. *JAMA, 323*(6), 509–510. https://doi.org/10.1001/jama.2019.21579

Mikalef, P., Lemmer, K., Schaefer, C., Ylinen, M., Fjørtoft, S. O., Torvatn, H. Y., & Niehaves, B. (2022). Enabling AI capabilities in government agencies: A study of determinants for European municipalities. *Government Information Quarterly, 39*(4), 101596. https://doi.org/10.1016/j.giq.2021.101596

Morley, J., & Floridi, L. (2019). The ethics of AI in health care: A mapping review. *Philosophy and Technology, 32*(4), 1–38. https://doi.org/10.1007/s13347-019-00362-5

Naamati Schneider, L. (2020). Strategic management as adaptation to changes in the ecosystems of public hospitals in Israel. *Israel Journal of Health Policy Research, 9*(1), 1–11. https://doi.org/10.1186/s13584-020-00424-y

Naamati-Schneider, L. (2022). Intraorganization conflicts of interest in hospitals adapting to a changing ecosystem. *Journal of Health Organization and Management, 36*(3), 265–278. https://doi.org/10.1108/JHOM-09-2021-0325

Naamati-Schneider, L. (2023). The effect of digitalization on service orientation and service perception among Israeli healthcare professionals: A qualitative study. *Digital Health, 9*. https://doi.org/10.1177/20552076231191892

Naamati-Schneider, L. (2024). Enhancing AI competence in health management: Students' experiences with ChatGPT as a learning Tool. *BMC Medical Education, 24*, 598. https://doi.org/10.1186/s12909-024-05595-9

Naamati-Schneider, L., & Alt, D. (2024). Beyond digital literacy: The era of AI-powered assistants and evolving user skills. *Education and Information Technologies*. https://doi.org/10.1007/s10639-024-12694-z

Naamati-Schneider, L., & Salvatore, F. P. (2022). Digital transformation in private dental clinics. In *Business advancement through technology Volume I: Markets and marketing in transition* (pp. 201–218). Springer International Publishing. https://doi.org/10.1007/978-3-031-07769-2_10

Naamati-Schneider, L., & Salvatore, F. P. (2023). Sustainability for healthcare organisations and systems: Cultivating strategy and governance processes for a better future. In D. Vrontis, A. Thrassou, L. Efthymiou, Y. Weber, M. R. Shams, & E. Tsoukatos (Eds.), Business for sustainability, Volume I. Palgrave studies in cross-disciplinary business research, in association with EuroMed academy of business. Palgrave Macmillan. https://doi.org/10.1007/978-3-031-37361-9_11

Olorunsogo, T., Adenyi, A. O., Okolo, C. A., & Babawarun, O. (2024). Ethical considerations in AI-enhanced medical decision support systems: A review. *World Journal of Advanced Engineering Technology and Sciences, 11*(1), 329–336. https://doi.org/10.30574/wjaets.2024.11.1.0061

Rahman, M., Victoros, E., Ernest, J., Davis, R., Shanjana, Y., & Islam, M. (2024). Impact of artificial intelligence (AI) technology in healthcare sector: A critical evaluation of both sides of the coin. *Clinical Pathology, 17*. https://doi.org/10.1177/2632010X241226887

Rong, G., Mendez, A., Assi, E. B., Zhao, B., & Sawan, M. (2020). Artificial intelligence in healthcare: Review and prediction case studies. *Engineering, 6*(3), 291–301. https://doi.org/10.1016/j.eng.2019.08.015

Ryan, J., & Sysko, J. (2007). The contingency of patient preferences for involvement in health decision making. *Health Care Management Review, 32*(1), 30–36. https://doi.org/10.1097/00004010-200701000-00005

Sallam, M. (2023). ChatGPT utility in healthcare education, research, and practice: Systematic review on the promising perspectives and valid concerns. *Healthcare, 11*(6), 887. https://doi.org/10.3390/healthcare11060887

Schwab, K. (2017). *The fourth industrial revolution*. Currency.

Sqalli, M. T., & Al-Thani, D. (2019). AI-supported health coaching model for patients with chronic diseases. In *2019 16th International Symposium on Wireless Communication Systems (ISWCS)* (pp. 452–456). IEEE. https://doi.org/10.1109/ISWCS.2019.8877113

Tekkeşin, A. İ. (2019). Artificial intelligence in healthcare. *Anatolian Journal of Cardiology, 22*(1), 8–9. https://doi.org/10.14744/AnatolJCardiol.2019.28

TerKonda, S. P., & Fish, E. M. (2023). Artificial intelligence viewed through the lens of state regulation. *Intelligence-Based Medicine*, 100088. https://doi.org/10.1016/j.ibmed.2023.100088

Thurzo, A., Strunga, M., Urban, R., Surovková, J., & Afrashtehfar, K. I. (2023). Impact of artificial intelligence on dental education: A review and guide for curriculum update. *Education in Science, 2023*(13), 150. https://doi.org/10.3390/educsci13020150

Veikkolainen, P., Tuovinen, T., Jarva, E., Tuomikoski, A. M., Männistö, M., Pääkkönen, J., Pihlajasalo, T., & Reponen, J. (2023). EHealth competence building for future doctors and nurses–Attitudes and capabilities. *International Journal of Medical Informatics, 169*, 104912. https://doi.org/10.1016/j.ijmedinf.2022.104912

Visan, A. I., & Negut, I. (2024). Integrating artificial intelligence for drug discovery in the context of revolutionizing drug delivery. *Life, 14*(2), 233. https://doi.org/10.3390/life14020233

Vyas, S., Bhargava, D., & Khan, S. (2023) Healthcare 4.0: A systematic review and its impact over conventional healthcare system. *Artificial Intelligence for Health 4.0: Challenges and Applications*, 1–17.

York, T. J., Raj, S., Ashdown, T., & Jones, G. (2023). Clinician and computer: A study on doctors' perceptions of artificial intelligence in skeletal radiography. *BMC Medical Education, 23*(1), 1–10. https://doi.org/10.1186/s12909-022-03976-6

Younis, H. A., Eisa, T. A. E., Nasser, M., Sahib, T. M., Noor, A. A., Alyasiri, O. M., Salisu, S., Hayder, I. M., & Younis, H. A. (2024). A systematic review and meta-analysis of artificial intelligence tools in medicine and healthcare: Applications, considerations, limitations, motivation and challenges. *Diagnostics, 14*(1), 109. https://doi.org/10.3390/diagnostics14010109

Yu, K. H., Beam, A. L., & Kohane, I. S. (2018). Artificial intelligence in healthcare. *Nature Biomedical Engineering, 2*(10), 719–731.

Zhang, W., Cai, M., Lee, H. J., Evans, R., Zhu, C., & Ming, C. (2024). AI in medical education: Global situation, effects and challenges. *Education and Information Technologies, 29*(4), 4611–4633. https://doi-org.mgs.hac.ac.il/10.1007/s10639-023-12009-8

Epilogue

Abstract Understanding the profound impacts of the VUCA world, alongside technological advancements and digital transformation, is essential for the future readiness of healthcare systems. This chapter, serving as the book's epilogue, underscores the critical need for competency-based education to prepare healthcare professionals for ongoing changes. By focusing on lifelong learning and adaptable management skills, it offers strategic recommendations for educators and healthcare leaders at macro, meso, and micro levels. These strategies aim to enhance healthcare systems' efficiency, quality, and stability, ensuring they are well-equipped to navigate future challenges and improve patient outcomes.

Introduction

In recent decades, technological advancements, automation, and the emergence of digital and virtual realms have brought about significant changes worldwide. Indeed, these transformations have given rise to the new concept of a VUCA world: a dynamic and unpredictable environment marked by Volatility, Uncertainty, Complexity, and Ambiguity. In this VUCA reality, the global economy has undergone profound shifts, fostering the need for creativity, innovation, and collaboration. To navigate this new landscape effectively, professionals across various domains must develop enhanced skills for solving unstructured problems and conducting thorough information analysis (Otter, 2019; World Economic Forum, 2015).

The pervasive influence of the VUCA world and the intricate challenges it presents have reverberated across different arenas, sectors and professions. As a result of the increasing complexity of organizational challenges in the current era, the VUCA world has had a major impact on management discourse, affecting all levels of healthcare systems worldwide: macro, meso, and micro (Cernega et al., 2024; Counte et al.,

L. Naamati-Schneider and D. Alt, *Technology and Competency-Oriented Learning*,
https://doi.org/10.1007/978-981-97-5771-8

2019; WHO, 2019; Worley & Jules, 2020). In addition to these global shifts, healthcare systems across the globe are confronted with major challenges and changes unique to their sector. The evolving healthcare ecosystem is affected by diverse factors, among them longer life expectancy, shifting demographics and geographic patterns, economic and political transformations, as well as the introduction of new regulations and reforms. These changes have contributed to a chronic and growing disparity between escalating healthcare expenditures and limited funding (Figueroa et al., 2019), exerting further pressure on the system. In extreme crisis situations, such as during the COVID-19 outbreak, this disparity becomes overwhelming, threatening the future sustainability, survival and stability of health systems worldwide (OECD, 2021).

Challenges and Directions Shaping the Future of Healthcare Systems

The aforementioned changes undoubtedly engender ongoing challenges. Projections of future increases in the demand for healthcare products and services along with forecasted resource allocations (WHO, 2019) point to a growing disparity between demand and budgets. This is exemplified by the expanding gap between countries' demographic growth rates and their average economic growth and GDP, coupled with the rising costs of health services and products. These disparities are anticipated to further magnify the inherent complexities of modern healthcare systems, yielding an uneven and unstable market (Counte et al., 2019).

The future is poised to witness the acceleration of various healthcare processes, including advancements in new technologies, remote treatment and analysis, applications, blockchain technologies, and the integration of artificial intelligence (AI) in treatment and service. Over the years, these developments have led to the rapid adoption of digital technologies within the healthcare industry (Naamati-Schneider, 2020, 2023; Naamati-Schneider & Salvatore, 2022, 2023). AI is set to be the next revolutionary technology that will transform the world as we know it. This innovative technique is accompanied by substantial challenges, barriers, and threats that require attention. The use of AI is anticipated to increase to the point that it will influence the structure of healthcare systems and organizations worldwide and transform the way people work and live (Ali et al., 2023; Manne & Kantheti, 2021; Wang & Preininger, 2019; York et al., 2023).

Moreover, the widespread adoption of technologies that provide remote service and care is poised to revolutionize the field of community medicine and home hospitalization. As these technologies gain momentum, increasing emphasis will be placed on improving the patient experience (Counte et al., 2019; Ghani, 2021). These anticipated changes are expected to enhance the efficiency and quality of services within the healthcare system. Nevertheless, they may also intensify the challenges faced by organizations and employees in coping with and adjusting to the evolving landscape (Bitkina et al., 2020; Wang & Preininger, 2019).

The future undoubtedly will bring numerous changes, difficulties, and challenges, some of which are still unknown to us. Hence, comprehensive systemic assessments are crucial for effectively navigating and adapting to these forthcoming changes. One of the most critical and challenging tasks at hand is to be able to comprehend and drive these changes proactively rather than being passively led by them. Indeed, a proactive approach is necessary to be able to understand and lead the transformative shifts needed to navigate these changes successfully.

To effectively implement these changes, we must acknowledge the significance of management's role and the importance of acquiring management skills specific to these transformative processes, as noted by this book. Such skills are essential and integral components of contemporary and future healthcare systems. Skills such as problem-solving, adaptability, creativity, flexible thinking, and innovation are indispensable for enabling teams, organizations, and entire systems to adapt to a dynamic market and unforeseen future conditions. Cultivating these skills and maintaining a continuous learning mindset are essential for navigating the ever-evolving healthcare landscape (Counte et al., 2019). Acknowledging and establishing the presence of managerial leadership roles within the healthcare system is crucial for leading these processes effectively. Healthcare leaders must be capable of managing strategic change and facilitating the assimilation of the organization's culture and environment while upholding ethical principles. To strengthen these capabilities, this volume innovates in the field of medical management education by emphasizing competency-based learning approaches and providing exemplary methods for this approach. This contribution is significant as it highlights the importance of developing specific competencies in healthcare managers and leaders, ensuring they are well-equipped to navigate the complexities of modern healthcare environments and drive continuous improvement. Such an approach is essential for facilitating effective adoption of change and for promoting seamless adaptation to anticipated transformations in healthcare systems worldwide. By embracing this approach, health professionals and patients will be able to navigate the ramifications of these changes more effectively, thus ensuring better outcomes for all stakeholders involved.

Throughout this book, we have highlighted the significance of an integrative approach in examining the evolution of healthcare organizations and professionals at three different levels: macro, meso, and micro. This approach emphasizes the transformative changes and challenges these systems currently face and underscores the critical skills necessary for effectively managing and adapting to these changes. Central to our narrative is the incorporation of the 21st Century Skills (21CS) taxonomy, which includes three core areas of competence—cognitive, intrapersonal, and interpersonal—and their applications across the three dimensions of the healthcare system.

Each chapter is tailored to a specific skill that is essential for healthcare managers. The chapters demonstrate how educators can cultivate competency-based learning methods and integrate technology and digital tools to enhance these skills. This comprehensive examination aids in understanding the complexities of healthcare systems and the essential competencies required for effective management.

Given the critical importance of adapting to the ever-evolving reality of change in healthcare as illustrated in this book, we recognize that the ability to adapt and enhance skills has become a crucial feature of the responsibilities of healthcare managers in the twenty-first century. With this in mind, in this section we delve more deeply into the practical aspects by offering recommendations tailored to a comprehensive range of key stakeholders within the healthcare system. Among these are educators in higher education institutions and those responsible for learning and development in healthcare organizations, as well as professionals engaged in healthcare practice and management. Our recommendations are categorized according to the three levels of the healthcare system: macro, meso, and micro. By addressing the needs and roles of these key groups at each level, we aim to offer valuable insights and strategies that are relevant across the entire healthcare system, from formal education settings to Continuing Professional Development (CPD). We also make recommendations for incorporating these insights into Workforce Development Programs to ensure that these strategies are not merely theoretical but also practically applicable in enhancing workplace competencies and outcomes.

Comprehensive Strategies: Practical Recommendations for Healthcare Education Improvement Across All System Levels

The macro level, highlights the importance of focusing on the entire healthcare system, with attention directed toward formulating policies, setting objectives, and establishing priorities. Hence, meta-leaders (McKimm et al., 2023) are needed at this level who will focus on fostering connectivity among diverse stakeholders in both intra- and inter-organizational settings. A holistic approach that goes beyond individual components is needed to serve as an effective driver for change across the entire system. This approach must foster collaborations and adopt a global perspective to facilitate extensive cooperation among professional organizations in the field, as highlighted by this book. By doing so, organizations can work collectively to set regulations and standards that establish the need for professional leaders in the field of medical management education.

This form of broad-based collaboration and activity should lead to the development of best practices, thus ensuring high-quality education and management across the healthcare industry. Accomplishing this goal requires a comprehensive plan that includes budgeting and strategic considerations for widespread medical and management education. Such a plan must incorporate collaboration among diverse global institutions operating at different levels of the healthcare system. By embracing this global holistic approach, organizations can foster a culture of ongoing learning, cooperation, and innovation that will yield meaningful and sustainable improvements in the healthcare sector. Implementing these plans requires nurturing leaders and educators in the health professions capable of training a large number of learners and qualified staff in both academic and healthcare service settings (McKimm et al., 2023).

This level of the healthcare system encompasses broader policies and system-wide standards. For this reason, this book emphasizes the need to incorporate ethical judgment, ethical leadership, and competencies related to Artificial Intelligence (AI). Additionally, adapting national healthcare policies and education standards to meet these evolving needs is essential. Uniform and standardized assimilation and integration of medical management education throughout different systems and organizations worldwide will promote more effective adoption of change and facilitate better adaptation. Such standardized practices will also help establish a common academic language to be used by the various higher institutions and medical schools involved in education and healthcare. The goal is to establish standardized and ongoing education, development and implementation at all managerial and organizational levels, from initial training to continuing professional development. By planning and integrating programs that focus on competency-based learning, the healthcare system can become sustainable and be prepared for whatever the future brings.

At the meso level, the focus shifts toward developing and implementing organizational and management strategies. These strategies encompass activities such as organizational adaptation, strategic managerial decision-making, budget management, procurement, streamlining work processes, and effective human resource management. To this end, as shown throughout this book, competency-based learning should be integrated by means of continuing education and enrichment activities for medical and management staff at all organizational levels. Educational initiatives and programs should be incorporated throughout the entire organization to ensure that healthcare professionals and managers receive comprehensive training and development opportunities. One possible option for effective implementation of this goal is to establish a unit dedicated to education and professional development within the organization. Such a unit can serve as an education hub responsible for designing and implementing a comprehensive curriculum to address the educational needs of all healthcare professions and disciplines within the organization. This hub for continuous development and training in relevant subjects will ensure that professionals acquire the latest knowledge and skills required in their respective fields. By establishing such an education hub, an organization can foster a culture of continuous learning and professional growth, ultimately enhancing the quality of healthcare delivery.

By implementing this approach, an organization can leverage the digital tools described in this book and can embrace technological advancements to facilitate effective professional training. Not only will such a comprehensive training program address technical skills; it will also focus on developing the intra-personal and interpersonal skills and competencies necessary to adjust to and keep pace with the rapidly transforming healthcare environment—an ability that is particularly important in the current AI era. Indeed, although AI technology is capable of automating specific tasks, it falls short when it comes to replicating intricate human capabilities such as empathy, creativity, and critical thinking—all of which are essential in the healthcare professions and in healthcare management. Recognizing this shortcoming of AI underscores the need to invest in fostering these qualities, skills and competencies through education, training, and practical experience. Focusing on areas such as effective communication, teamwork, leadership, adaptability, emotional intelligence, and ethical decision-making will enable healthcare professionals to utilize AI as a valuable tool rather than as a substitute for their unique strengths. Using AI effectively necessitates a mixture of skills, with a strong focus on mastering the prompting techniques that are crucial for guiding AI systems effectively and ensuring relevant and accurate outputs.

Moreover, establishing an educational hub that encompasses training for management, leadership, and professional development will enable organizations to underscore their dynamic and adaptive nature. The educational hub initiative will help shape an organizational culture that fosters adaptive change processes and lifelong learning skills, together with 21st Century Skills that will facilitate adaptation to the changing environment. Furthermore, by emphasizing the creation of educational hubs, organizations can establish a framework for cultivating agility among the workforce. These hubs will serve as adaptive tools that can equip employees with the knowledge and skills necessary to react and respond swiftly to the ever-changing environment. By fostering a culture of continuous learning and providing resources for ongoing education and development, organizations can empower their employees to engage in proactive adaptation and innovation, enabling them to thrive in a rapidly evolving ecosystem.

At the micro level, the focus further shifts to the individual level of the directors and the medical staff. Due to the evolving needs, demands and technological advancements of a rapidly changing world, today's knowledge and skills may become obsolete tomorrow. The fulcrum of this book is the increasingly evident need to focus on cultivating a set of lifelong learning skills. At this level, the focus must extend beyond the mere development of skills before embarking on a career and during the period of professional activity. Instead, medical professionals and managers must become lifelong learners and taking personal responsibility for learning throughout their careers. For this to happen, individuals must be equipped with the ongoing ability to acquire new knowledge, adapt to emerging technologies, and engage in continuous personal and professional development. By internalizing the importance of lifelong learning, individuals can remain agile, embrace emerging technologies, and continue to be relevant in an ever-evolving landscape.

The above discussion underscores the benefits of starting early to foster these skills. Given the rapid pace of change and technological advances in today's world, individuals must be trained to adapt continuously in order to remain relevant in their fields. Indeed, these skills and competencies must be developed and fostered from the early stages of their professional journey. In this regard, this book suggests that higher education institutions and medical schools, offering programs in healthcare practice and management, have a significant role to play. They must take the lead in integrating the acquisition of lifelong learning skills and an updated set of 21st Century Skills within their curricula and educational settings. To this end, they must incorporate pedagogical approaches and tools that promote the three core areas of competence—cognitive, intra-personal and interpersonal—by means of critical thinking, problem-solving, adaptability, collaboration, self-regulation, and the integration of emerging technologies. By doing so they will equip students with the tools and mindset necessary for continuous skill development throughout their careers. This proactive approach will enable future healthcare professionals and managers to navigate the dynamic landscape of the healthcare industry, enabling them to effectively embrace and lead transformative changes in the healthcare sector.

Indeed, the dynamically evolving healthcare sector is marked by a growing need to develop and integrate a competency-based pedagogical approach to professional healthcare and management education. Adopting such a paradigm is critical to the development of professionals who can lead the transformative processes necessary for survival in the diverse, technologically challenging and ever-changing environment of twenty-first century healthcare.

As shown throughout this volume, this shift to a competency-based pedagogical approach in healthcare management education should permeate all levels of the system and be accompanied by comprehensive planning, budgeting and strategic implementation. The transition should range from the early stages of education to the level of ongoing professional development in order to ensure consistent integration of this paradigm through all the stages of educational and professional development. Such a comprehensive approach is essential to produce managers and professionals who are well equipped to meet the multiple challenges of modern healthcare.

This book raises the call upon researchers, educators, healthcare administrators and key stakeholders worldwide to adopt and advance this competency-centered pedagogical approach. Indeed, this approach is essential to sustain healthcare management as a discipline characterized by agility and rapid adaptability. Only through such a concerted effort will we be able to navigate the complexities and constant change marking today's healthcare landscape.

References

Ali, O., Abdelbaki, W., Shrestha, A., Elbasi, E., Alryalat, M. A. A., & Dwivedi, Y. K. (2023). A systematic literature review of artificial intelligence in the healthcare sector: Benefits, challenges, methodologies, and functionalities. *Journal of Innovation and Knowledge*, *8*(1), 100333. https://doi.org/10.1016/j.jik.2023.100333

Bitkina, O. V., Kim, H. K., & Park, J. (2020). Usability and user experience of medical devices: An overview of the current state, analysis methodologies, and future challenges. *International Journal of Industrial Ergonomics*, *76*, 102932. https://doi.org/10.1016/j.ergon.2020.102932

Cernega, A., Nicolescu, D. N., Meleşcanu Imre, M., Ripszky Totan, A., Arsene, A. L., Şerban, R. S., Perpelea, A. C., Nedea, M. I., & Pițuru, S. M. (2024). Volatility, uncertainty, complexity, and ambiguity (VUCA) n healthcare. *Healthcare, 12*(7), 773. https://doi.org/10.3390/healthcare12070773

Counte, M. A., Howard, S. W., Chang, L., & Aaronson, W. (2019). Global advances in value-based payment and their implications for global health management education, development, and practice. *Frontiers in Public Health, 6*, 379. https://doi.org/10.3389/fpubh.2018.00379

Figueroa, C. A., Harrison, R., Chauhan, A., & Meyer, L. (2019). Priorities and challenges for health leadership and workforce management globally: A rapid review. *BMC Health Services Research, 19*(1), 1–11. https://doi.org/10.1186/s12913-019-4080-7

Ghani, S. (2018). The future of healthcare: Turning challenges into opportunities. *Health Management, 18*(3).

Gupta, R., Tanwar, S., Tyagi, S., & Kumar, N. (2019). Tactile-internet-based telesurgery system for healthcare 4.0: An architecture, research challenges, and future directions. *IEEE Network, 33*(6), 22–29.

Manne, R., & Kantheti, S. C. (2021). Application of artificial intelligence in healthcare: Chances and challenges. *Current Journal of Applied Science and Technology, 40*(6), 78–89. https://doi.org/10.9734/cjast/2021/v40i631320

McKimm, J., & O'Sullivan, H. (2016). When I say… leadership. *Medical Education, 50*(9), 896–897. https://doi.org/10.1111/medu.13119

McKimm, J., Ramani, S., Forrest, K., Bishop, J., Findyartini, A., Mills, C., Hassanien, M., Al-Hayani, A., Jones, P., Nadarajah, V. D., & Radu, G. (2023). Adaptive leadership during challenging times: Effective strategies for health professions educators: AMEE Guide No. 148. *Medical Teacher*, 1–11. https://doi.org/10.1080/0142159X.2022.2057288

Naamati Schneider, L. (2020). Strategic management as an adaptation to changes in the ecosystems of public hospitals in Israel. *Israel Journal of Health Policy Research 9,* 65. https://doi.org/10.1186/s13584-020-00424-y

Naamati-Schneider, L. (2022). Intra-organisation conflicts of interest in hospitals adapting to a changing ecosystem. *Journal of Health Organisation and Management*. https://doi.org/10.1108/jhom-09-2021-0325

Naamati-Schneider, L. (2023). The effect of digitalization on service orientation and service perception among Israeli healthcare professionals: A qualitative study. *Digital Health, 9*. https://doi.org/10.1177/20552076231191892

Naamati-Schneider, L., & Salvatore, F. P. (2022). Digital Transformation in Private Dental Clinics. In *Business advancement through technology volume I: Markets and marketing in transition* (pp. 201–218). Springer International Publishing. https://doi.org/10.1007/978-3-031-07769-2_10

Naamati-Schneider, L., & Salvatore, F. P. (2023). Sustainability for healthcare organisations and systems: Cultivating strategy and governance processes for a better future. In *Business for sustainability* (Vol. I, pp. 227–248). Palgrave Studies in Cross-disciplinary Business Research. Palgrave Macmillan. https://doi.org/10.1007/978-3-031-37361-9_11

Otter, K. (2019). Developing leadership: innovation, adaptability and integration in large-scale health care organizations. *Experten führen: Modelle, Ideen und Praktiken für die Organisations- und Führungsentwicklung*, 179–192. https://doi.org/10.1007/978-3-658-23028-9_10

Siyal, A. A., Junejo, A. Z., Zawish, M., Ahmed, K., Khalil, A., & Soursou, G. (2019). Applications of blockchain technology in medicine and healthcare: Challenges and future perspectives. *Cryptography, 3*(1), 3. https://doi.org/10.3390/cryptography3010003

Wang, F., & Preininger, A. (2019). AI in health: State of the art, challenges, and future directions. *Yearbook of Medical Informatics, 28*(01), 016–026.

WHO. (2019). *World Health Organisation: Universal health coverage*. Retrieved from https://www.who.int/news-room/fact-sheets/detail/universal-health-coverage-(uhc). June, 2022.

World Economic Forum. (2015). *New vision for education: Unlocking the potential of technology*. World Economic Forum.

Worley, C.G., & Jules, C. (2020). COVID-19's uncomfortable revelations about agile and sustainable organizations in a VUCA world. *Journal in Applied Behavioral Science, 56*(3), 279–283. https://doi.org/10.1177/0021886320936263

York, T. J., Raj, S., Ashdown, T., & Jones, G. (2023). Clinician and computer: A study on doctors' perceptions of artificial intelligence in skeletal radiography. *BMC Medical Education, 23*(1), 1–10. https://doi.org/10.1186/s12909-022-03976-6

GPSR Compliance

The European Union's (EU) General Product Safety Regulation (GPSR) is a set of rules that requires consumer products to be safe and our obligations to ensure this.

If you have any concerns about our products, you can contact us on ProductSafety@springernature.com

In case Publisher is established outside the EU, the EU authorized representative is:

Springer Nature Customer Service Center GmbH
Europaplatz 3
69115 Heidelberg, Germany

The manufacturer's authorised representative in the EU is Springer
Nature Customer Service Centre GmbH, Europaplatz 3, 69115 Heidelberg,
Germany. If you have any concerns regarding our products, please
contact ProductSafety@springernature.com

Printed and bound by CPI Group (UK) Ltd, Croydon, CR0 4YY
01/10/2026
02225859-0002